CANCER...there's hope

This book is available to you without charge with the belief that it offers you methods to improve the quality of your life and increase your chances of successfully fighting cancer. After you have read the book, please give it to another cancer patient. If you are unable to do this, please give it to a library or minister so that they may loan it to someone it can help.

We would appreciate hearing your feelings after you read this book. Drop us a note. We care about you!

The Cancer Hot Line
Annette and Richard Bloch
4410 Main Street
Kansas City, MO 64111
(816)-932-8453
(816)-WE BUILD

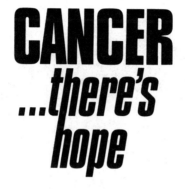

RICHARD AND ANNETTE BLOCH

CANCER
...there's
hope

Published by
R.A. Bloch Cancer Foundation, Inc.
4410 Main Street
Kansas City, Missouri 64111
816-932-8453
A not-for-profit corporation

First printing - April 1982
Second printing - March 1983
Third printing - April 1987
Fourth printing - December 1988

Printed in the United States

Book designed by Jack O'Neal

contents

preface

In 1978, Richard Bloch, co-founder and honorary chairman of the board of H&R Block, Inc., contracted cancer. With the help of his wife, Annette, and the doctors who said he could lick the disease, and with a stubborn determination to survive, Bloch waged a bitter, painful, two-year war on the insidious disease.

Today, he is cured.

So dramatic was his fight and recovery that Bloch and his wife have decided to spend their lives helping to convince others that they too can cope with cancer.

The purpose of this book is to advise cancer patients, their relatives and friends what could be involved and what some of their options are. It is also to advise doctors and other professionals what reactions there could be to statements or treatments. The more knowledge we have about this dreaded disease, the better we can help ourselves and others cope.

dedication

This book is dedicated to our three daughters, Barbara, Nancy and Linda, whose love, support and devotion gave me the will and the desire to live.

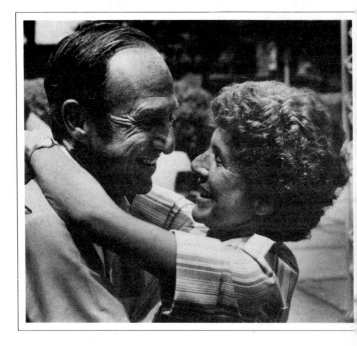

chapter 1

Understanding what lies ahead

On March 28, 1978, the doctor told me that I had a malignancy. My lung cancer was inoperable. I should get my estate in order.

Two years later, the doctors told me I was totally cured. I have no more chance of a recurrence of lung cancer than anyone else on the street.

This book is being written for the benefit of any individual who has been diagnosed as having cancer or who has a friend or relative who has cancer. It will attempt to explain different stages and treatments of the disease as seen through the eyes of one who has gone through it.

It is not a series of medical stories. Everything in it is from personal experience. These are my feelings about, or my understanding of, what was happening.

It is my hope that there is something here that everyone will be able to to relate to. Nothing is intended to be used as a comparison, because every case of cancer is different. Not only are there different types of cancers, but they are in different places, happening to people of different ages, of different backgrounds and of different strengths and weaknesses. Each case of cancer is as unique as a fingerprint.

The reader should be able to better understand and empathize with what the person with a malignancy is going through and what that person can do to help himself. It is to show how important is good medical attention, how vital is prompt action, and how fundamental is a positive mental attitude.

Cancer is the uncontrolled growth of cells. Cancer cells are extremely small. One million cancer cells would be the size of the head of a pin. One billion, that is 1,000 million, would be the size of a small marble. These cells are weaker than healthy cells, but gain their strength because they multiply so readily.

There are six possible fundamental treatments or therapies used to cure cancer. They may be used individually or in any combination. They are:

• Surgery. The simple act of cutting out the tumor.

- Radiation therapy. Killing cancer cells with X rays.
- Chemotherapy. The use of chemicals to kill cancer cells.
- Immunization therapy. The use of chemicals to activate the body's own immune system to kill cancer cells.
- Heat therapy. Killing cancer cells by localized heat.
- Psychotherapy. The controlled use of the mind to kill cancer cells and stir up the immune system to kill cancer cells.

Surgery, radiation and heat therapy are localized approaches. They deal with a specific locale of cancer and are effective against large masses. On the other hand, chemotherapy, immunization therapy and psychotherapy are systemic approaches. That is, they go throughout the entire system. They are possibly less effective against a large localized mass, but will destroy cancer cells in small quantities throughout the body. For this reason, it is generally best to use one or more of the localized treatments to eliminate the mass and then follow up with one or more of the systemic therapies to ensure that all traces of cancer have been destroyed.

Since cancer multiplies geometrically (one cancer cell divides into two, two divide into four, four into eight, and so on), it is obvious why it is so important to discover it as early as possible and then treat it immediately. Don't ever look back and criticize yourself because you didn't discover it earlier. Once it is discovered, it is important to treat it properly and promptly. One day's delay could mean the difference between life and death.

Radiation and certain chemicals can be given to the body only in limited amounts. Certain kinds of surgery cannot be repeated. For example, you can only remove one lung one time; you cannot have the second lung removed and live. Therefore, it is often critical that the cancer be totally cured the first time, as there is no hope of successfully treating certain kinds of recurrences. An interesting related example was explained to me by a doctor. They found that a certain type of leukemia always went into remission on its own. It then recurred and was fatal. But by taking bone marrow from the patient during this universal remission, freezing it and then injecting it back into the same patient when the leukemia recurred, the doctors usually cured the patient.

In my personal case, I attribute my recovery to five factors:

- The total support and devotion of my wife and my children; they gave me the will to fight.

- Finding the right teams of doctors. I must be grateful, not only to the doctors who properly treated me, but to all those who devoted themselves to discovering the treatments that were used on me.

- Positive mental attitude. Once the initial shock was over, I knew I had to make it and would do anything to accomplish this.

- Luck. The fact that the tumor formed around a nerve drove me to seek additional opinions.

- Faith in God. My prayers and the prayers of so many others which meant so much to me had to be a factor.

chapter 2

First recognition

My bout with cancer started the first week of November 1977. We had rented a villa in Acapulco for five weeks. It was during our first week there that I noticed the signs of an oncoming stiff neck. I attributed this to either the vigor of playing platform tennis every morning or to the window air-conditioner in our bedroom.

I never mentioned it to my wife; I assumed that it would be gone within a week. On the contrary, it did not disappear, and it gradually increased over our five-week stay.

On my return to Kansas City, I called my family doctor and made an appointment to see him the next morning. He took an X ray of my shoulder and said it was strictly a muscular problem.

I told him how relieved I was. But, for some reason, this pain in my shoulder reminded me of a pain that my uncle complained about before he died of cancer. Told this, the doctor took three more X rays of my shoulder and said he could guarantee that it wasn't cancer. He also said the soreness should be gone within thirty days. This was December 15. It also was the first time I told my wife about my problem.

We went to Florida for the month of January. The pain was still there. It got worse and started slipping down my arm. On my return to Kansas City, I made an appointment with an orthopedic surgeon in the same building as my physician. He immediately sent for the X rays that had been taken. He said they had X-rayed the wrong part of my body. He took four X rays of my neck and showed me that the problem was arthritis in my neck that was rubbing a nerve causing the pain in my shoulder and arm. This made a great deal of sense, and I told him that I had been worried about cancer. He too reassured me that my fears were unfounded and that the pain should go away in another month.

We returned to Florida. But instead of disappearing, the pain increased to the point where my arm began tingling and was partly numb. Often I was unable to grip with my right hand.

Again, returning to Kansas City on March 27, 1978, I called another orthopedic surgeon. He had been highly recommended. At this point I wanted to determine the cause of my pain. Immédiately on explaining my problem, he said that he was not the man for me to see. He recommended that I go to a neurosurgeon. I gave him a brief explanation on the phone and hoped that he would see me that week. Instead, the neurosurgeon said he wanted to see me within the hour at the emergency room at Research Hospital.

My wife and I met him there. He asked me to turn my head back and forth, and he promptly assured me it was not arthritis. He asked me how much I smoked. I said I didn't like that question; I knew full well that it meant that all my previous fears could be correct.

I am grateful to this man. He was the first doctor to recognize the problem, and he acted speedily to verify it. He arranged for me to be at another hospital at seven-thirty the next morning, to take an electronic test of my right arm to determine the extent and location of the nerve damage, and to do a chest X ray. That X ray revealed a large mass in my right shoulder on the upper part of my lung; it appeared to be very serious. Immediately a bone scan of my entire body was taken, and it indicated that I had a tumor. A biopsy was scheduled for the next morning to determine whether it was malignant.

While I was under a general anesthetic, my wife and three daughters sat patiently, not really believing what was happening. After the biopsy, while I was in the recovery room, the surgeon and his assistant came to the waiting room to tell the results to my family. He was quite blunt; he came right out and told my wife and daughers that I had lung cancer, that it was very serious, and that there was possibly, at the most, a 30 percent chance of recovery.

What a cruel and unnecessary way to break the news. Honesty is important, but there are less cruel ways of getting the message across. My family wept with anguish and disbelief. They composed themselves and started discussing with my brother Henry and his wife what possible alternatives there were.

Meanwhile, when I regained consciousness in the recovery room, the surgeon was there. His words to me were, "It is malignant. It is inoperable. If I were you, I would get my estate in order."

I asked if there was any treatment other than surgery possible. He answered that they could give me radiation therapy, but it would not do me any good and only make me sicker. I asked whether there was anywhere else I could go, and he said he would send me anywhere I wanted to go, but no one knew any more than he did.

At this point, they wheeled me out of the recovery room. My wife was standing there waiting for me. We looked at each other. I broke down and cried. My wife, by this time, had regained her strength and told me, "We are going to lick this thing together."

My feelings at that moment were of total disbelief. The doctors had to be talking about someone else. I was a healthy, happy, fifty-two-year-old man, and things like this always happened to the other guy. My wife and I had been married thirty-one years, had three wonderful daughters, two sons-in-law, four grandchildren, and a successful business. All in all, I had just too much to live for. I wanted to know more, but I didn't know what or whom to ask.

I did not even know what this disease called cancer really was. My mind was so blown that I could not recall that I had ever known anyone who had cancer. I had momentarily forgotten that my uncle had died from it, and less than eight years before we had watched my wife's sister painfully die from it. We wanted help, but we didn't know where to turn.

That night, a friend, Buddy Greenbaum, whose wife had recently been a victim of cancer, called. He had just heard about my problem and, without even asking me, had called his wife's doctor in Houston. He told him about me, and the doctor said he would wait at his home for my immediate call.

I called the Houston physician. This was Wednesday night. He told me to come to Houston on a plane Thursday and start tests Friday at 8 A.M. I said that I would prefer waiting until Monday, as I had some personal and business affairs to attend to. The doctor informed me that the clinic was closed over the weekend. Since time was of the essence; if I was not in Houston Thursday night, the doctor said, he would not treat me.

Thursday morning at six-thirty I was in my beautiful office for possibly—no, *probably,* according to the doctor—my last time. I loved my office, not only because of what it is, but what it represents. Physically, it is very contemporary, done in shades of brown, rust, orange and chrome. The accessories are mementos from various trips to the Near East and Far East.

My office represented something that had been built from scratch. My brother Henry and I had started a business from our imagination. We had over 8,000 offices around the world preparing income tax returns. I thought of all the people along the way who had helped us and had become extremely successful. I thought of all the individuals we had helped. That's what my office represented, and I was leaving it to catch a 5 P.M. flight for Houston that afternoon.

I had come to the office to get my papers in order, but I just sat and stared and thought. My entire wonderful life passed before me. I had enjoyed every minute of it and tried to help everyone I met along the way. I had no regrets. I was not afraid to die. I just hated to leave when I was having such a great time.

I opened a desk drawer and took out a Christmas card that my daughter Barbara wrote for me in 1976. In part it said:

. . . And then I pictured you at play—a 50-year-old little boy with a mischievous gleam in your eye as you sailed the boat toward the beach to ride the waves.

You take such delight in everything you do!

And I said Thank God for your spirit.

And I thought about the determination with which you do everything—sometimes bordering on stubbornness!—but displaying a stamina that I must admire.

And I said Thank God for your strength . . . In standing firm you stand so tall.

And I thought about how you have conveyed to me the importance of giving . . . not by words, but by setting an example. I was so proud that you donated to Breakthrough House. Not only was it a substantial and needed gift, but it was acknowledgment and approval of something I was doing. That gesture meant more to me than you know. And I thanked God for your generosity."

After reading the card, I knew I had to make it. I would not quit. I would fight this with Annette until we beat it. If Houston did not turn out to be the right place, we would keep looking. I needed my family, and they needed me too much to throw in the towel.

That evening we checked into the Anderson-Mayfair Hotel, carrying our X rays, slides, and numerous reports. We had come for an indefinite period. The feeling of not knowing whether we'd be leaving in a day, a week, a month, or never, was very difficult.

Early the next morning we went to the clinic to register me as an outpatient. From the time we saw the sign M.D. Anderson Tumor Clinic, we felt good. In the indoctrination, we were shown a film on what we could expect, and when we realized that this institution every day treated 1,200 patients who suffered from some form of cancer, we knew we were in the right hands.

In addition to this confidence, the cheerful attitude of all personnel did a great deal to allay the fear and terror of hearing the word *cancer.* Later on, we would learn that a substantial share of the cure of cancer comes in the waiting room, talking with other patients who have been cured or are being treated.

After the orientation, we met the doctor, who is a professor of medicine and head of the section of immunization therapy. He explained that I would be given numerous tests on Friday. The clinic would be closed on Saturday and Sunday, during which time the results of the tests would be analyzed. He would meet with me Monday morning.

It was to be one of the most thorough and exhausting days of examinations I've ever been through, including brain scan, liver scan and tomograms, and culminating in a very painful bone-marrow test. At the time, I was willing to let them do anything they wanted, because I felt that each test they gave me meant a slight chance of survival over the prospect of doom that had been forecast in Kansas City.

I finished the tests at 5 P.M. We had the weekend to ourselves. When death is knocking on your door, what do you do? Where do you go? We had no desire to face family and friends in our depressed state of mind. This would merely have evoked sympathy and would have caused unnecessary suffering on both sides.

We decided then to run away to a little apartment we had in Fort Lauderdale, Florida. It was quite a weekend. My wife and I were deeply immersed in our thoughts and questions, many of which went unspoken. We sat alone and silent for long periods of time.

Our mutual love was a little speed boat named "After Taxes." The first morning we went to a store and got some wine and cheese and packed a picnic lunch. We went out on the boat, no goal, just cruising around and thinking and trying to talk.

We thought of all the trips we had taken together. Annette thought that she had never done anything without me. If she didn't have me, she'd never want to come down here.

Here we were, both young, and we had the most incredible family. Three fabulous daughters, two sons-in-law and one on the way, four grandchildren. We loved to travel with our children. If something happened to me, this all would stop.

And here we were facing death.

On our cruise to nowhere this Saturday, we found a tiny island, no more than fifty feet across. It was in the middle of the city, where the New River bends away from the Intercoastal Waterway, but at least 150 feet from the nearest shore. A lot of birds were there. The sand was white. We saw this and, on the spur of the moment, beached the boat.

We got out of the boat and sat there and just started talking. We couldn't believe this was happening. Was it real? This didn't happen to people we know.

We decided then and there that we had to beat it. We talked about how much we loved each other. I had to get well.

Annette sensed my fear. I really love life and have always enjoyed every moment of it. I've always seen the good in others. Annette kids me that I have never found the hole in the doughnut. I wasn't ready for this life to stop. We looked at each other and knew that I had to make it. We just had to lick it. Annette picked up a stick and drew a big heart in the sand the way kids do. She put our initials in it and the date, and scribbled, "We Shall Return."

We drank some wine and talked. We got back into the boat, drove off and anchored out in the water where we wouldn't see people. We talked some more. But a lot of the time we didn't say a word. We sat and thought.

chapter 3

Starting down
the road to recovery

 Monday morning, April 3, 1978, we returned to Houston and met with my doctor. He advised us that he and several other doctors had reviewed the results of my tests and discussed my case at great length.

His exact words were: "Dick, you are a very sick boy. We are going to make you a lot sicker, but we are going to cure you. We are going to cure you so that you can work for cancer."

Melodramatic? I guess so. But hope is the one ingredient that every human clings to. It gives us a reason to live, to fight. If I could struggle to the end of this grim path, survive the radiation and chemotherapy, I told myself, I would devote my life to helping others stricken as I was.

We were truly elated; these were the first positive words and first ray of hope we had been

given. As much as we wanted to, it was difficult to fully believe, comprehend and accept.

The doctor explained that the treatments I
would be receiving had never been done before
in this exact sequence. I would be given two
weeks of radiation therapy, immediately fol-
lowed by one week of chemotherapy. I would
be allowed to recuperate and regain my
strength. Surgery would then remove the dis-
eased area, and immunization therapy would
follow immediately. After recuperating from
this, I would receive one year of chemotherapy.

The logic behind this was explained to me.
Cancer cells are extremely small. One million
cancer cells are the size of the head of a pin.
One billion cancer cells are the size of a small
marble one centimeter in diameter. Cancer
cells can be killed more easily than healthy
cells. The radiation therapy that I would receive would kill precisely 72 percent of my
cancer cells each day. Therefore, if I started off
with 100 billion cancer cells, after the first day
I would only have 28 billion left. After the
tenth day, I would only have 296,000 left.

Chemotherapy, on the other hand, can do
very little against a large, massive cancer, but
is excellent at killing isolated, individual can-

cer cells. Therefore, after the two weeks of radiation, the week of chemotherapy should be extremely effective against the relatively few cancer cells left. Also, a big problem in cancer is that since the cells are so small, they tend to break off from the main tumor and lodge themselves in other parts of the body. The brain and the liver both tend to strain blood, which is why cancers so often metastasize, or spread, there. The chemotherapy before surgery was to prevent the cancer from metastasizing somewhere else while I was recuperating from radiation and lung surgery.

As for the immunization therapy, it is predicated on the belief that everyone has an immune system that constantly kills cancer cells. Through some sort of weakness, this immune system may let down and allow the cancer cells to grow. Obviously, since I did have cancer, I had a flaw in my immune system.

Research has found that people who have had tuberculosis rarely get lung cancer. On this premise, I was to be given tuberculosis after surgery to stimulate my immune system and keep me from getting lung cancer again after recovery.

The year of chemotherapy was to take away

any chance of recurrence. While the odds were great that I would be completely free of cancer, the likelihood that a recurrence would be fatal made any odds too risky.

chapter 4

Radiation therapy

Tuesday morning my wife and I wound our way to the area in which the hospital does radiation therapy on the chest. We had to pass through the head and neck radiation department. There were sixty chairs lined up against two walls that ran the length of the room, and every chair was taken. The people were bald, shaved, with red lines painted on their heads and necks. It was like walking through Dante's Inferno. It was like another world. They looked like people from outer space. They looked like a whole different civilization. I couldn't look. I didn't want to. It made my skin crawl.

This was not a comforting sight for someone like me who had no idea what to expect.

I was ushered into a small auditorium with possibly twenty-five doctors in the audience. I sat on the podium with the radiologist; my X rays were displayed as my case was discussed. I had no comprehension of the meaning of the

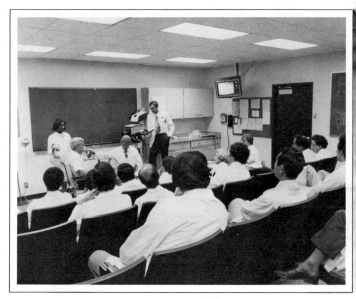

Planning Radiation Therapy

questions or answers, the terms were so technical. However, I did realize that they were formulating the best possible treatment for my individual case. I felt very good about this.

I was shown what appeared to be a magnificent X-ray machine and was told to lie on the table. It was explained that this machine was just a dummy with no internal working parts. It was used to set up my future treatments and to save time on the expensive real equipment. The doctor took a Magic Marker, measured, and then put a dot on me. Then another dot and another dot. Then he connected the dots. What was he doing? There was no knife. Just a Magic Marker. I rolled over and he did the same thing on my back. He used a ruler and was very precise about it. He put different things on my chest, blocks and the like. He would find the right one and trace around it. The reason for this was so that each treatment would be given in the same location.

When the radiologist finished marking me up I looked like one of those sketches of a side of beef, the shank section here, the brisket there, the sirloin, the T-bone, the flank, and so on.

It took him maybe an hour to measure me.

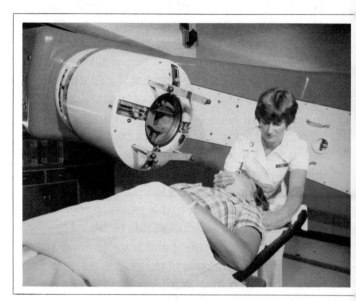

Nurse positioning patient for radiation therapy

It was all calculated by computer. There was a terminal in the room.

I was unhappy that I had not been fore-warned that I would not be allowed to take a shower for two weeks so as not to wash away the red lines.

All the calculations were made, and the computer was programmed to give me my treatment. With trepidation, I went into one of the two rooms containing the real working equipment. The machines looked awesome. They were operated automatically by a com-puter controlled by an individual watching me on television outside the room. It took a nurse probably two minutes to get me properly posi-tioned on each side, with lead shields sitting on my chest or back to keep the rays away from sensitive organs. The treatment itself was less than forty seconds on each side. The sensation was exactly the same as having your picture taken — absolutely nothing. I was amazed; I had expected much worse.

The doctor had warned me that there would be no feeling to the treatment, but fourteen days after the last treatment I would have the worst sore throat I had ever had.

Each morning at eight o'clock I came down

to this department for my treatment, a process that took about five minutes. I had the rest of the day free. During this time, my wife and I did a great deal of reading of everything we could find about cancer. In the Houston paper was an article about a clinic in Fort Worth. It was run by a husband and wife named Simonton. He was a radiologist, and she was a psychologist. Together they founded this clinic based on the premise that the mind can stimulate the immune system and help cure cancer. Being doctors, they believe in medical treatment first and foremost. However, they have developed methods of strong positive thinking that have produced an amazing track record.

As I remember it, their statistics of a test group of terminal cancer patients with no known medical treatment available showed that after two years approximately 10 percent were in complete remission, another 10 percent were improved and a third 10 percent had their cancer stabilized. To us, this was quite a revelation. We decided that if the M.D. Anderson Tumor Clinic told me they could not help me, then we would go to the Simonton clinic. In the meantime, I would practice my own interpretation of their positive thinking and imaging.

This meant to me to picture in my mind my cancer. I pictured an ugly, black mass in my shoulder that looked something like a big glob of tar. However, it was constantly in motion like a turbulent thundercloud. In my mind I kept hitting this glob with my fist and breaking little pieces off and throwing them away. I kept picturing each treatment dissolving a little more of this glob. I kept concentrating on this type of disintegration intently. Possibly the fact that I had been told the radiation would kill 72 percent of these cancer cells each day helped this concentration.

chapter 5

Chemotherapy

During the two weeks of my radiation therapy, Annette did quite a bit of reading about the chemotherapy that I would be facing. Supposedly, there was a great deal of nausea and discomfort connected with most powerful drugs. She had read that marijuana could be used to alleviate a great deal of this discomfort and had been legalized in certain states for this purpose. She talked to the doctor, who confirmed this, but he said that Texas was not one of the states. She was determined to try anything to help make my treatment a little easier. However, I was adamant about not smoking marijuana cigarettes. I had gone through such a traumatic experience in giving up smoking two years before that I was determined not to do anything that could undo this effort.

I knew nothing about marijuana. I had never in my life smoked it. I had never tried it in any form.

The doctor said that if we had a way of getting some, well, it might help. One of our daughters found some. We decided that a marijuana brownie would be it. A doctor called a doctor friend of his in California and asked what the formula was for making magic brownies. We got his recipe. Annette and our daughter stayed up until 1 A.M. before my first chemotherapy treatment, trying to make a batch of brownies. She had to clean the stuff, but she didn't know what she was doing. She decided to put a lot of thick icing on it to disguise the taste of the marijuana. Annette told me later, "I thought if there was a lot of icing on it, you wouldn't taste anything." It was so rich, it was terrible.

At seven the next morning, I reported to the chemotherapy ward. The bed I was assigned to was in a room with a dozen beds, six perpendicular to each long wall, with about five feet between them. There were curtains that could be drawn around a bed for privacy, but they were kept open most of the time. The bright lights made resting difficult and revealed the need for painting and repairs. A bottle of fluid hanging on an IV stand next to each bed was connected by a rubber tube to each patient. The moans and groans along with the sounds of retching and the smell made it seem like a snake pit. When I walked into it, the thought of an extended period of this made my knees weak and my stomach squeamish before even starting.

A lovely nurse patiently explained what I would be going through. She gave us, in writing, a detailed description of each of the four drugs I would be receiving, including what each was, what each would accomplish, the schedule by which each would be given to me and what effects each drug would have.

Chemotherapy is technically therapy by the use of chemicals. When a person takes two aspirins, he is taking a form of chemotherapy. While I was to receive chemotherapy from 7 A.M. until 7 P.M. some days and 11 P.M. other days, most of the time I was receiving water or a saline solution intravenously. The chemicals are so strong that it is necessary to flush them through your system. A great deal of water, therefore, is given before and after the chemicals.

With the explanations out of the way, it came time to start this dreaded treatment. Before starting, I ate a quarter of a "special" brownie that my wife and daughter Nancy had so meticulously prepared. I took one large bite, tasted it, forced myself to swallow it and promptly vomited. The icing was so rich and the marijuana tasted so awful, that I can honestly say that this was worse than any of the chemotherapy that ensued. For months, I would wake up with nightmares of that taste. To this day, just the thought of that brownie makes my stomach queasy. So much for my one and only experience with marijuana!

Chemotherapy started. Annette and Nancy sat by my side throughout these four long days. Watching me and my fellow patients continuously getting sick and suffering was very distressing for them. They felt so helpless in not being able to ease my discomfort. At night, I was so weak that it took the two of them to get me to the car and to the hotel across the street.

On the brighter side of things, practicing the positive mental attitude I had read about, I was grateful for this sickness. If these drugs could make this big strong body so violently ill, think what they would be doing to those weak little cancer cells. It really helped me think my cancer away.

The discomfort itself could actually be compared to the sickness you have from drinking too much. When I was younger and had had too much to drink on New Year's Eve, I felt the same way. The difference is that this went on for four days and left me continuously weaker. One of the great times of my life was to be leaving that hell hole on Friday night and flying back to my home in Kansas City, even though I had to be taken to the airplane in a wheelchair.

Little did I know what I had in store for me. Even though the chemotherapy had completely destroyed my appetite, I was looking forward to three weeks of rest and relaxation with no treatments. That is how long I had to recuperate before surgery.

As weak as I was, the next few days I got progressively weaker. Chemotherapy had completely distorted my sense of taste and smell. My favorite foods no longer had any appeal to me. Certain odors that I had been faintly aware of, and had tolerated for years, suddenly became intolerable. Betty, our cook, would fix something in the kitchen, and even though I was in our bedroom at the opposite end of the house, I couldn't stand the smell. We had a stand of dried flowers, and I couldn't take their odor. I kept asking why Betty was burning the coffee. I would take one sip of it, and it was the worst-tasting stuff.

I guess I got kind of mean about things. I was very demanding. I didn't realize that my taste was distorted. I thought the foods weren't being cooked right, and I got very angry about it.

I was always cold. If it was 75 degrees, I would be cold. I'd turn off the air-conditioner, and everybody else would suffer. I didn't know whether my blood was flowing, or what was going on.

One of the incredible things about the whole experience is how precise the doctors were in knowing exactly what was going to happen to me. You'd think it was guesswork, but it wasn't. They said I would have a sore throat a certain number of days after I got home. I did. It was the worst sore throat anyone ever had. It was like a charley horse you get in your leg, except this was a cramp in my throat. There was no way anything was going to get down my throat. Betty babied me for days. She would make things like a soft-boiled egg and give me a half teaspoonful. I'd some-

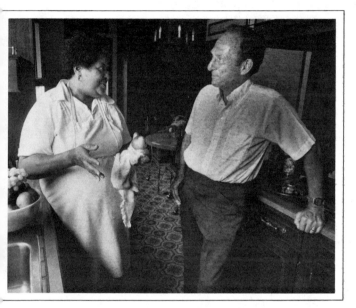

Betty Logan, the cook, talking with Dick

how get it down, and she'd clap her hands and yell, "Hallelujah!"

At first, I couldn't even swallow a drop of water. Betty and Annette tried baby food and canned food supplements. For two days, I couldn't take anything. Sometimes Annette had to literally jam food down my throat. I knew that Annette wanted me to eat, and I knew it was important for me to eat, and I was upset because I couldn't. I was losing weight.

I knew that if the radiation had done this to the healthy cells of my throat, it really must have played havoc with the weaker cancer cells.

Slowly but surely the pain and nausea subsided and my strength started returning. However, my strength did not come like Samson's. Along with the return of my strength came the loss of my hair.

Though this had been foretold, I was totally unprepared for the reality of being transformed into a Yul Brynner or a Telly Savalas. It started off with a few hairs clinging to my comb, then more appeared on my pillow each morning, until finally it came out in huge clumps. Within a week, I did not have a hair on my entire body — including eyebrows, arms, legs, everywhere. Surprisingly enough, it did not bother me nearly as much as it bothered everyone else who had to look at me.

My youngest daughter, Linda, was engaged to get married five weeks after my surgery. She was thoughtful enough to volunteer to postpone the date, but I was determined to let nothing change her plans. My wife asked me as a favor to have a toupee made, thinking it would make me feel better about my appearance. I went along with the idea, knowing it would make her happy; I truly didn't care. Even though I was to be bald for the next year, the *only* time I wore the toupee was during the wedding festivities.

The doctors' forecast on my recuperation period was incredibly accurate. I felt physically better each day. The night I arrived in Houston, I felt so terrific that I took my wife and daughters out for a fun evening on the town. We found the nicest restaurant in Houston. I don't know how many bottles of wine the four of us drank. We didn't know if we would ever be able to eat and drink like this again. We went back to the hotel, and the four of us got in our king-sized bed together. Barbara, thirty, Nancy, twenty-seven, and the two of us. We giggled and laughed. We were like four little kids. We hugged and kissed. It was like trying to erase from our minds any thought of the impending surgery and possible consequences. We succeeded.

chapter 6

To surgery

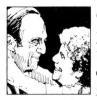

On Monday, I entered the hospital for numerous tests. One of these was under a giant machine that measured my breathing capacity, section by section. The purpose supposedly was to advise the doctor how much of my lungs could be removed and still allow me to live. I was told that this was one of two machines like it in the United States and its results were figured by a computer in Minneapolis. I thought of all the people who have lung surgery without the aid of numerous tests.

It was ten-thirty that night before the doctor could get me scheduled for a tomogram. This took a separate X ray of my chest vertically each third of an inch from my neck to my stomach by computer. The doctor wanted the best possible information in advance on what he would find when he opened me up.

The day before surgery, an orderly came into my hospital room with a kit and asked my

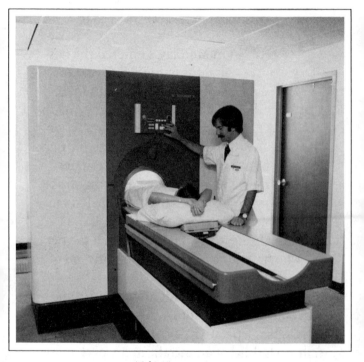

Taking a tomogram

family to leave so that he could "prep" me for surgery. I was scared of what he was going to do to me. All he did was shave my stomach and back. A simple explanation, instead of technical terms, could have avoided the apprehension.

There was another unnecessary experience when I asked one of the assisting surgeons how much use of my right arm I could expect to lose. He answered that he did not know—which is where he should have left it. He then went on to volunteer that I should realize that I was facing the worst possible kind of surgery and that I had everything to lose and nothing to gain. This was not the type of surgery to repair or improve something. This was to go in and remove anything they saw that was cancerous, short of killing me.

He said, "You cannot come out any better than you went in. You can only come out worse. We are going to get rid of the cancer, and wherever we see cancer we have to take it out. We have no idea how far it is. If we have to, we'll take off your whole shoulder. You could come out without a right arm."

He had no reason to be that grotesque. That's what was on my mind the night before surgery—the awful, negative things that he said. I suppose doctors think they're preparing us for the worst. Where is the possible bene-fit? How can a cancer victim think positively if this is what he hears?

The anticipated morning of May 16 was here. As I was being wheeled down to surgery, my last recollection in my drugged state was the secure and warm feeling of seeing my wife, three daughters, sons-in-law, two broth-ers and my sister-in-law all there together and sharing this burden with me. I felt truly blessed!

chapter 7

Recuperation

The entire family spent the long, grueling time in the waiting room. My wife and children alternately sat and paced, wrapped up in their own thoughts. Hovering over them was the possibility of never seeing me alive again. My wife was very positive, however, and kept repeating that I just had to make it.

Annette later said, "I don't think I will ever forget in my whole life the call we got to come down to the surgery floor. The surgery was over. The surgeon wanted to talk to us. At the same time my heart started pounding, and I was panicked, because I didn't know what he was going to tell us. He was either going to tell me that Dick had made it, or that it was the end. We had to go into a waiting room. Everyone was quiet. I never stopped pacing or praying. I was like an animal in a cage. I had my fingers crossed. We had to wait for the surgeon. It seemed forever, but it was maybe ten minutes. When he walked into the room, I really think my heart stopped.

"Time literally stood still. Everyone was afraid to breathe a word. I walked up to him, and he stood there, suddenly with a smile, and said, 'Why are you looking so unhappy? Everything is fine.' My head started spinning. We couldn't believe it. He sat down and told us everything."

He had removed the top lobe of the right lung, two ribs and part of a third, and certain nerves in my right shoulder. He told them the tumor had shrunk so much that he had been able to remove every trace of it. The unusual thing was that the biopsy, after removal, showed no sign of any living malignant cells. Everyone cried from happiness, and my wife took everyone out for dinner to celebrate.

When I finally awoke the next morning, I knew all was well, because I saw that everyone was smiling. The surgeon explained that two tubes in my side connected to a pump were for drainage. He further explained that the nerves that he had removed from my shoulder would prevent my side from perspiring and would also make me unable to play tennis. With that statement, I looked him straight in the eye

and said, "Oh yes, I will play tennis again."
At any rate, it would have been a small price
to pay to have gotten rid of the cancer.

My recovery started very normally. I had to
do long, tiring lung exercises each day. They
explained that pain would impede my recovery, and I was given pain pills regularly. After
a few days, I was given BCG through one of
the tubes in my side directly into my pleural
cavity. BCG is a drug for immunization
therapy. It causes an illness that is similar to
tuberculosis; it is easily cured, and it stirs up
the immune system against a recurrence of
lung cancer. Sure enough, within a few days,
I had a very high fever—around 105 degrees.
They started me on a pill a day for thirty days.
At the end of that time, I was all cured of the
"TB."

I spent three weeks in the hospital. My three
daughters, Barbara, Nancy and Linda, took
weekly turns being with Annette so that she
was never exposed to this ordeal alone. Each
room on my floor was a private room with an
extra sofa bed for a family member to sleep
on, if desired. This reemphasizes M.D. Anderson's belief that cancer is an illness needing
family support and the importance of having

a caring friend or relative with the patient at all times.

The hospital at M.D. Anderson is only a 400-bed hospital. Yet there are six full-time ministers on duty. Even though I would not classify myself as an extremely religious person, the daily visit by one of the ministers meant a great deal to me.

A retired Houston rabbi, Hyman Schachtel, whom we had met in Kansas City, also called on me every day in the hospital. His visits and his warmth were very meaningful and gave me strength.

Get-well cards, letters, flowers and phone calls started pouring in. Each one was treasured. I heard from friends I had long lost contact with. I can't emphasize enough the importance of letting someone who has cancer know that you are thinking of him and really care.

Probably the most meaningful thing to me was the people who said they'd say a prayer for me. A casual friend in Kansas City told me he said a prayer for me every morning. I figured that, with my prayers and with all these people saying prayers for me, I had to get well.

Two weeks after surgery, the realization of the loss of the use of my right hand and arm hit me. I could not even hold a pencil, let alone write. They sent me to see a physical therapist. He again did an electronic test on my right arm to determine the extent of the nerve damage. He marked about eight red X's at various points on my right arm. He gave me a machine to use that would send electric shocks when these X's were touched with electrodes to regenerate the nerves in my arm. If you have ever shocked yourself, you would know what this feels like. My wife had to do it to me for five seconds and rest for five seconds, for 2 ½ hours twice a day. We were elated on the last day, when the shocks caused the respective finger to quiver.

Three weeks after surgery, I returned to my home in Kansas City, weak, bald, looking as if I had aged ten years, fearful of anyone getting near my sensitive right side, but—alive! The doctor said I would be home to walk my daughter down the aisle.

As in everything else he said, he was right.

chapter 8

The ups and downs of treatment

Thank goodness, I was home at last and able to think about getting ready for Linda's wedding.

I was bald as an eagle. Not only was there no hair on my head, but there was not a single hair on my entire body. I was down to 145 pounds. I looked awful. Annette wanted me, as a favor to her, to get a toupee. "Honey," I told Annette, "for you I'll do anything."

Annette thought the toupee would make me feel better. She thought that I looked old, when I wasn't really old. She felt that if I looked good, I would feel better. We ordered a $300 toupee. When it came in and they put it on me, I had never had that much hair in my life. Annette sat next to me and told the barber exactly how she wanted it cut, while he did it.

So he cut and trimmed it. When we got home, Annette wanted me to try it on again for her. "That's still too much hair," she said. So we went back, and the barber cut more off, exactly to her specifications. He charged us $20, but it made Annette happy. The week before the wedding Annette asked me to try the toupee on again. Again she said, "It's still too much." Back to the same barber, and another $20 later I could wear it to the wedding. Here it is, a toupee, and it's not growing, and it still has to get three haircuts.

I never wore it again after the wedding. Everybody who saw me after the wedding, without the toupee, said they liked my looks better without it.

At the wedding, I walked Linda down the aisle, and I had the first dance with her, just as we had planned before the cancer treatments.

At the end of June, I had to go to Houston for a physical examination. I was feeling substantially stronger. I assumed that it would be a routine test and I would be back home the next night. The doctor said my lung had filled with fluid, and he put me back in the hospital. That was a low blow—just when I felt things were going so well, to have a setback like this.

He wanted to put the tubes back in my side

to drain the fluid. I was really feeling too good to go through this kind of pain and discomfort, and I talked him into waiting a few days. After lying in my hospital bed for four days doing absolutely nothing, I had an X ray the morning of July 5. The congestion had cleared itself up and I was free to go home.

On the one hand, I was so happy and excited, and on the other hand, I was angry that they had kept me in the hospital over the Fourth of July for no reason at all.

My wife was extremely worried that I had suddenly turned into an old man, a fact that I could not see in myself. Besides my physical appearance, being totally hairless, gaunt and sallow, I moved like an old man. Every move I made was very slow, including shuffling at an octogenarian's gait. My wife kept telling me to stand up straight and lift my feet when I walked. She didn't realize that it was more comfortable for me to hold my right arm motionless, to constantly protect my right side, and to slide my feet, one after another, in a stooped position. She tried to convince me that I was still young and that I should act it. At times I resented her relentless urging, but later I was grateful that she had kept it up. Finally she turned to the doctor for assistance. The lecture he gave me was not to be forgotten; starting then and there, I made a concerted effort to act my age, stand straight, lift my feet, and smile.

Simultaneously, something new was to happen to me. In my childhood I was greatly overweight, and all my adult life I have been on a diet. In the past thirty years I had been able to go from 190 pounds to 165. Candy bars and milk shakes were something to be remembered from childhood. Midnight snacks were for someone else. For thirty years it had been three meals a day, no sweets, no snacks. Now I was suddenly at 145 pounds.

My doctor explained that weight loss could be an indication of cancer and conversely, in order to prove that I was rid of cancer, he wanted me to put on weight. This would have been a dream a year before, but after my sore throat, my marijuana brownies, my surgery and chemotherapy, regular eating, to say nothing of excessive eating, was not a pleasant thought. However, I made up my mind that this was part of my cure and I was going to do it.

Some days for lunch I would stop by a pancake house and have pancakes covered with butter and floating in syrup. It didn't take very long. At 155 I asked the doctor to let me stop, as this was where I wanted to be. Permission denied. At 165 I again asked and was again denied. Finally, at 170, I was allowed to go back to normal eating.

It took a year of strict adherence to conservative eating to get back to 165. It seems like such a long way to 155, but at least I'm here to keep working on it.

Then came my biggest problem. I did not want to take any more chemotherapy. It was uncomfortable, unpleasant and weakening. I felt that these powerful drugs could cause problems with various organs of my body later on in life. I felt that I was cured, not only because of all the treatment I had had, but particularly because no trace of living cancer cells was found after my surgery. So why punish my body further?

The doctor said that I was going to take chemotherapy. My wife insisted that I do what the doctor ordered, since he had already saved my life.

I had asked everybody I saw about taking chemotherapy. During my recuperation, one of the assistant surgeons said that he had been

there during the entire operation. He saw that
they had removed every trace of the cancer and
that, if it were he, he wouldn't go through the
ordeal of chemotherapy.

While I was home, a friend of many years
visited me on my patio. She had had her lung
removed because of cancer the previous year,
and her surgeon had told her that she was totally cured and did not need chemotherapy.

Another friend had come down with lung
cancer two weeks after me. His surgeon removed his lung, gave him a clean bill of
health and advised that chemotherapy was
not necessary.

I related these experiences to my doctor, and
his vehement answer was, ''Dick, nobody
asked you. You are going to have chemotherapy.''

My wife's feeling about this was that one
should do the best for oneself and never look
back and say, ''I wish I had,'' after it's too late.
When I think how small cancer cells are, they
are obviously not individually visible to the
naked eye. Therefore, any doctor who says he
removed all the cancer really means he removed all the cancer he could see. There is no
way he could possibly see a few isolated cancer
cells in another part of the body, such as the

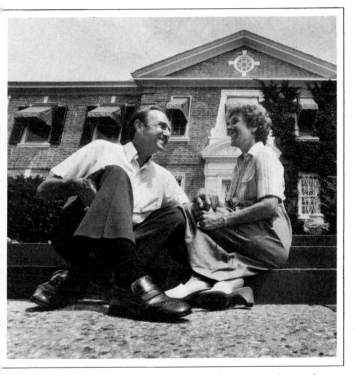

Dick and his wife, Annette, sit on the steps in front of their home

other lung, the liver or the brain.

Within a few months after her visit to my patio, my friend developed cancer in her other lung. Obviously, surgery and strenuous treatment were no longer an option, since she had only one lung. Soon afterward she died. The same thing happened to my other friend. In the past two years, two more acquaintances were pronounced cured of cancer after a lung was surgically removed. Both had been told they didn't need chemotherapy. Both died of cancer in the other lung.

I am not a doctor. I am not trying to say that everyone who gets cancer needs chemotherapy. I am trying to say that if I were told I did not need chemotherapy, I would want an oncologist (cancer specialist) to verify that statement. In many cancers, there is only one chance to beat it. If you don't go all the way the first time, there may not be a second chance.

In order to avoid excessive trips to Houston, my Texas doctor arranged for a young oncologist in Kansas City to give me my chemotherapy treatments. Not only was it convenient to have a local source for treatment, but it was valuable to have a local authoritative source for answers to the questions that would arise. These two doctors were in constant contact about my case.

The basic chemotherapy treatment was to be given one week each month with three weeks following to recuperate. I used to say it was a diabolical scheme — every month they let you get well just to make you sick again.

I think some of the drugs I took were interesting, even though many of them today could be totally out of date. One drug was supposedly the oldest chemotherapy drug around — 5 F.U. I understood it was more than twenty years old. It was given to me intravenously along with the other drugs during my week of treatment. The following week, I would have to go to the doctor's office for an infusion of this drug. Infusion is merely a shot of it in a vein of my arm. I got to the point where I could take this infusion on my way to the office. It didn't bother me at all.

By contrast, one of the drugs I took, Adriamycin, was nicknamed "the Red Devil." This drug had been discovered ten years before, had been tested for two years, and had been used only for eight years. Even though very few people have ever heard of it, the doctor told me that this drug saves more lives every year than the Salk polio vaccine. This is the drug that makes you so violently ill and also causes the loss of hair. Interestingly enough, after my treatments a way was discovered to avoid losing your hair. It is simply to wear an icepack on your head during the time you are receiving Adriamycin and for a few minutes thereafter. However, this is not always advisable, nor does it always work.

A third drug was Cysplatinum, apparently made from the metal platinum and extremely expensive. After a few treatments, the pharmaceutical company stopped making it. Another company started, but it was off the market several months until the FDA approved the new manufacturer's process. I was unhappy at being denied this drug for those few months. I felt that, as long as I was going through such discomfort, there should be the best odds of success.

The fourth drug was Cytoxin.

Along with my philosophy of positive thinking, I welcomed this terrible ordeal each month. I knew that if it was making me so violently ill, it had to be killing the last traces of any cancer cells which may have spread throughout my body.

But, let me say that this year was not all bad. The last week in July, my wife and I were able to take a one-week business trip to Bermuda. My November treatment was given a week early, and the December treatment a week late to enable me to spend a month in Acapulco.

For some reason, my December treatment affected me adversely. I got quite weak and developed a moderate fever. We left between Christmas and New Year's to take our three daughters and three sons-in-law on a Caribbean cruise. On the ship, I seemed to be getting continuously weaker. At our second port, Grand Cayman, we called my doctor in Houston. He told me to go to a hospital, have a blood test, and call back immediately with the results. We did, and he wouldn't believe the results were so bad. He insisted that I have another test and call back. As much as I hate to have blood drawn, we complied with his wishes. The second results verified the initial findings. He explained to me on the telephone that my blood was in such a condition that if I came in contact with any germ, I would have no ability to fight it and would be dead within twenty-four hours.

The eight of us just sat and stared at one another in disbelief. He insisted that I not get back on the ship, but immediately fly anywhere in the United States where there would be facilities to treat me. He talked to the head doctor and explained the situation.

But every flight was completely sold out. The doctor had to use his influence, due to the severity of the situation, to have two people removed from the next flight out so we could fly to Florida. My children went back to the ship and hastily packed our clothes.

Fortunately and coincidently, my Kansas City oncologist was vacationing in Fort Lauderdale, and he came to see me immediately on my arrival. I had to stay in bed for two weeks, except for going to the hospital every other day for blood tests. Each time I would call my doctor in Houston with the results. During the second week, he said that the most recent test had to be wrong, and I should have the hospital check it. I called the hospital, and they verified the results. The doctor wanted me to immediately fly to Houston for a platelet transfusion. I said I was feeling too good for there to be any problem. He then told me that if I started bleeding, it would not stop, and he asked if my gums didn't bleed when I brushed my teeth. I said no. He compromised and allowed me to have another blood test the next morning. Sure enough, this proved that the hospital had made a mistake the previous day. Oh, the highs and lows of this strange disease.

The end of January, we stopped in Houston on our way from Florida to Kansas City for my routine quarterly examination. I was feeling fine, and I knew that everything was A-OK. All the tests were administered the first day, and the second day we visited with the doctor before catching our flight home. He seemed particularly perturbed and kept us waiting quite a while.

The doctor then confronted us with the fact that my X ray had shown a substantial mass in my shoulder. Numerous doctors had reviewed this and could not determine whether it was scar tissue or a new tumor. He wanted me to go immediately to the hospital to be admitted for a needle biopsy.

My wife and I looked at each other in disbelief. This just couldn't be happening — espe-

cially since everything had been going so well.
We were completely undone by the whole
thing. I had taken every recommended treatment. We had played the game as cautiously
as we knew how. I was feeling too well. We
were to be secure in our own home in a couple
of hours — yet, here we were, in the hospital
awaiting surgery. I, myself, had seen the mass
in the X ray.

I was ready to cry. I told my wife I could not
go through this whole thing all over again. In
her strength, she told me we could and we
would, if we had to.

The needle biopsy did not show any malignancy. This did not necessarily mean that
there was no tumor, as it is possible to miss the
tumor or miss the cancerous cells.

The next day we were released to go home
with the provision that I would get a chest
X ray each two weeks to monitor any change.
This indicated to me how fast cancer can grow.
These X rays showed no changes.

The last day of March, we again returned to
Houston for a routine examination. The next
morning in our conference with the doctor, he
mentioned it had been a year since I started
treatment. He asked my weight, did some

calculations, and told me that I had taken all the chemicals my body could tolerate. I was finished with chemotherapy. What a happy day! Those were the most wonderful words I had ever heard in my life.

I would continue to come to Houston for semi-annual checkups. During my visit on May 1, 1980, the doctor said, "Dick, I won't be seeing you professionally any more." I didn't know what to make of this statement. He explained that with the type of cancer I had, if there was no recurrence within two years, I had no more chance of getting it back than anybody anywhere. As a matter of fact, I probably had less chance of a recurrence of lung cancer because of the immunization therapy.

Furthermore, in my case, it had been twenty-five months, and each month is important. Some cancers are watched for five years, some for ten years and some for fifteen years, but in my case, the crucial period was two years.

This entire conversation came as a total surprise for me. I thought I'd be going to Houston for years with the constant threat of recurrence. For the second time in my life, I thought the doctor was talking to someone else or about someone else. I could not believe or hope that I would ever hear the words that I was cured. There surely is a Good Lord above.

chapter 9

Mind over matter

I had never been a pill taker. The Houston surgeon insisted that I take a pain pill every four hours after surgery. That was five a day, each containing one grain of codeine. He explained that the surgery had left a great deal of scar tissue in my shoulder. A little pain medication taken regularly, before pain and the resulting tension started, would keep me relatively free of pain and allow me to heal faster.

Again, I am not a pill taker. Twice—once in July on our way to Bermuda and a second time in August at home—I tried to break the habit. Both times, on the second day, the pain was intolerable and I had to go back to using the codeine.

On my next regular visit to Houston, the doctor recommended that I see the M.D. Anderson Tumor Clinic staff psychologist. We visited him in the afternoon of my departure. I explained that I didn't believe in psychiatrists or psychologists. I felt that I was an intelligent individual and was able to control my thoughts without help.

He started off by saying that since I was leaving that afternoon, he would be unable to treat me, so he would like to tell me a story. Subconsciously, this established my confidence in him, since he could have no personal motive.

He told me to picture myself walking across Main Street with a tremendously sore leg. Each step means excruciating pain. I am barely able to hop. In the middle of Main Street, I glance up and suddenly see a huge truck coming at me at 60 mph. What happens? Suddenly, I have no pain and I am easily able to run the rest of the way across the street to avoid being hit by the truck. When I reach the curb and stop, the pain is back in full force. What does this prove? The mind is capable of turning off pain if it wants to.

He recommended that when we got back to Kansas City, we find a psychologist who treats pain.

My wife made numerous phone calls and

did a great deal of research. She made an appointment for me with a doctor. He explained that pain was a combination of two factors: tension and physical hurt. If I could learn to relax and get rid of tension, the pain would be less severe. I always thought of myself as a very relaxed person, but I did not know the true meaning of the word.

On the first visit, he taught me how to relax. I was to lie or sit in a comfortable position, close my eyes and say to myself that each part of the body is relaxed. For example, my forehead is relaxed, my eyebrows are relaxed, my eyes are relaxed, and so forth down to the toes. Then I was to picture myself floating into an absolutely quiet room and from there floating into a beautiful garden with a quiet lake and the sun streaming through the trees and then lying in the grass surrounded by the aroma of fresh flowers.

Believe me, after this you are really relaxed. I was to do this every morning when I woke up and every night before I went to bed. Usually when I went to bed, I never got out of the first room, as I fell asleep from being so relaxed.

On my second visit a week later, the doctor attempted to use hypnosis to stop the pain. It

did not work. The third week he tried again
without success.

On the fourth week, after relaxing me, he
asked me to think of the most beautiful
thought I could imagine and tell him what it
was. I said it was my wife's love for me. He
then said that my body was filling with my
wife's love for me and repeated that it was
completely filling my entire body. I took my
good left hand and placed it on the left side of
my chest and rubbed it across to my right
shoulder forcing my wife's love for me into the
right shoulder and all the pain out. It worked.

From the time I left the doctor's office that
day, I never took another pain pill. Whenever
my shoulder started hurting, I thought of my
wife's love for me and forced it up into my
right shoulder and instantly the pain was gone.

As I have mentioned, friends are wonderful
to have. It was through such a friend, Alfred
Lighton, that I met a physical therapist who
was to do much to change my life.

After surgery, I had been left with no muscular control in my right hand and arm. Even
after hours of shock treatment, I could not
move a finger on its own or raise my arm
above my shoulder. With the help of my other

hand, I could only slightly bend each finger or move my wrist. I had made the idle boast to the Houston surgeon that I would play tennis again in spite of his saying otherwise.

The M.D. Anderson physical therapist cautioned that I could atrophy and permanently lose the use of my muscles if I didn't attend to it right away. That scared me into wasting no time making inquiries.

The physical therapist we found in Kansas City came to my house first thing in the morning for an hour, three times a week, to work with me. Her method was superb. She never touched me. She made me want to do things myself and do them until they hurt. She was a tough, but gentle and patient woman. After she left each time, I was to repeat the therapy several times before her return.

The first two weeks were spent just trying to bend the fingers of my right hand. Each time, I'd say there was no possibility that a finger would bend any more, she'd have me compare it to the other hand. I would then continue to painfully press further. She would strap weights on my arm, stand me in front of a mirror, and make me raise my arm. After a month, we cut her visits down to once a week because she said I had the drive and desire and could practice on my own.

One week, without her knowledge and to surprise her, I took my tennis racket out to the court. I was able to hold it but not raise it. I would stand in front of the backboard for thirty minutes at a time, hitting tennis balls against the backboard from three or four feet away with my racket like a pendulum. After a few weeks of this, I was gradually able to move further back, raise my racket higher and grip it tighter.

After another month, she dismissed me. She said I was one of her outstanding successes. I had achieved total mobility of my arm, wrist and fingers. The strength, as much as possible, would come back in time.

I realized, though, that I was not as strong and would never be so on the tennis court. Therefore, I would have to make up for it with accuracy and strategy. I got a larger racket and practiced placing shots; I now believe my game is as good today as it ever was, if not a shade better.

After surgery the doctor told me that because he had to remove nerves from my shoulder, my right side would no longer perspire. I

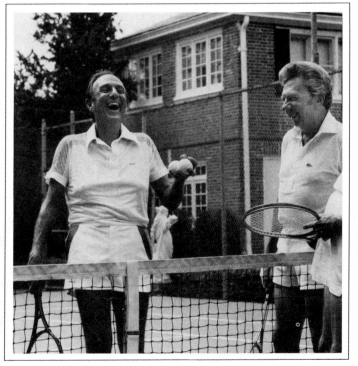

Dick and his brother, Leon, on the court

would have to keep my right arm covered whenever I was in the sun because it would burn without perspiration being able to cool it. Some two years later, completely to his surprise and ours, my arm suddenly started perspiring again. What a weird thing to get excited about.

No one shaking hands with me or looking at me would ever know that my right arm was impaired. Today, the inside of my arm down through my little finger is numb, and I do not have the strength to open some twist-off jar caps. These trivial things are a small price to pay for having conquered cancer.

chapter 10

Creating hope—
the Hot Line

 On the flight home from Houston on May 1, 1980, the words that the doctor had used on April 3, 1978, rang loud in my ears. "Dick, you are a very sick boy. We are going to make you a lot sicker, but we are going to cure you. We are going to cure you, so that you can work for cancer."

He was as good as his word. Here I was, going home, cured. It was at this moment that I decided to dedicate the rest of my life to helping people with cancer. The big questions were where and how.

I went through the important factors. They included early recognition of cancer, eliminating the causes of cancer, discovering new treatments for cancer, creating immunity from cancer, treating and curing cancer. Where could I fit in best?

Since at that time the U.S. government

donated about $1 billion a year toward the fight against cancer, and the American Cancer Society raised nearly $200 million a year, I knew that any financial contribution I made would not be meaningful. Besides, I really wanted to give of myself.

I remembered an old adage that you can write a better story if you write it from personal experience. Therefore, my forte had to lie in the treatment and cure of cancer. The other four factors are best handled by qualified scientists and doctors. I had been through the treatment and cure of cancer, and no one knew more about my thoughts, feelings, emotions and trauma than I did.

My mind went back to the day when the surgeon told me I had a malignancy. My wife and I were numb, disbelieving and tormented by questions, with no place to turn to for answers. I realized that I was not unique, that most people must have these same feelings. Furthermore, there must be many other cured or recovering cancer patients who would be eager to help. It would be wonderful to set up a group of lay volunteers who have or have had cancer and would be willing to talk with newly diagnosed victims.

If I could only have seen a person who had recovered from lung cancer, it would have meant everything to me. Even if he never said a word, I would know that if he could do it, I could do it too. These thoughts developed into the Cancer Hot Line.

I arranged a luncheon with the executive director of Human Rescue, Inc., a non profit crisis intervention telephone service. My thought in contacting him was that Human Rescue already had telephone lines with volunteers to answer them. If we could use their facilities, all we would need in order to have the Hot Line in operation would be the cancer volunteers. He listened to the concept of the Hot Line, liked it, and offered the use of his resources.

Since we had Human Rescue to answer the phone, all we needed was volunteers and training for them. I had lunch with a psychiatrist, and he, with the help of a social worker, agreed to plan and give the training.

Jerry Smith, a retired Kansas City businessman and philanthropist, headed up the Cancer Hot Line and arranged to use Central Methodist Church as headquarters for training.

The key to the success of the Cancer Hot

Line is publicity, to make people so aware that when a malignancy is diagnosed and their minds are completely disoriented, they will still recall the publicity and call the Cancer Hot Line. Furthermore, this publicity must be directed toward people who have absolutely no interest in it. It must be directed to healthy people who "know" they will never get cancer and do not want to hear about it.

I felt confident that once the publicity broke, we would have an abundance of former cancer patients as volunteers. However, we needed a few screened and trained volunteers, so that we could handle the calls that came in from the initial publicity.

Through my acquaintances and others in the program, a nucleus of volunteers was gathered and trained in early August. There was extended discussion on the amount of training to be given. Some people wanted all volunteers to attend four sessions, to be taught all terms relating to cancer, descriptions of various types of cancer and so on. I persevered and won out in that volunteers were taught what not to say. Everything else must come from their personal experience. It has since proved to be the right way.

The Cancer Hot Line is a reality. It is a group of lay volunteers who have or have had cancer and are available to talk on the telephone and possibly visit a newly diagnosed cancer patient or potential cancer patient. The victim calls the Cancer Hot Line number (in Kansas City, it is (816) 932-8453) and gives certain relevant information, including name, age, sex, address, phone number and type of cancer. A volunteer who has had the same type of cancer and most nearly matches the sex, age and location, will contact the victim within fifteen minutes, if possible.

The purposes of this contact are many. It immediately shows the victim that his type of cancer is not necessarily fatal and can be treated. It gives him a lay friend who can commiserate with him. It allows him to ask all his unanswered questions. The answers are in simple language, they are from personal experience and not from textbooks, and there is no pressure or fear of taking up a professional's time.

The volunteer is screened and trained to never give a prognosis or medical advice. He is to serve as a sounding board, tell of personal experiences that imply hope, and do two con-

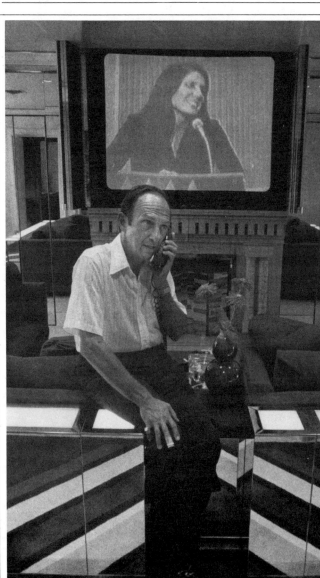

Richard, taking a Hot Line call at home

crete things: first, see that the patient is getting prompt, proper and thorough medical treatment, and, if there is the slightest doubt about this or about the patient receiving a favorable prognosis, the volunteer will refer the patient to the Cancer Management Center; second, the volunteer is to see that the patient reads this book and *Fighting Cancer*.

The volunteer may, if he desires and thinks it wise, be in regular and frequent contact with the patient to be certain that the patient is doing what is best for himself.

When I explained the hot-line concept to a friend, he said that friends of cancer patients also need it. He had a good friend and law partner with a malignancy. The partner called and told him from the doctor's office and never returned to his law office. My friend could never bring himself to visit, because he did not know what to say or how to act. He did not see him again until the funeral. So, the Cancer Hot Line program has been expanded to include not only families of patients, but also friends.

I do not profess to have any medical knowledge or ability. Everything I know about cancer is from personal experience, reading or hearing. Some of the questions I personally have heard on the Hot Line have been shocking to my untrained ears. They show the dire need for this service in every community.

Could one of these comments apply to you, your friend, or your relative?

"My doctor says I am malignant and to come back in six months to see how the tumor has progressed before planning treatment." (He went to an oncologist and is currently being treated, with a favorable prognosis.)

"The plastic surgeon who is giving me chemotherapy for my lung cancer, which he says is inoperable, has told me I am dying." (He came to the panel. The doctors recommended a series of different therapies. His present prognosis is favorable.)

The absolute coincidence of a patient telling me that he is going to be given chemotherapy by a doctor who says he won't make it—the same doctor who told me, personally, sixty days before, that he was a hematologist. He

*would be happy to serve on our panel
if we had a case of leukemia, but he
knew nothing about other types of cancer. (This patient agreed to see an oncologist.)*

*A woman in Florida who wanted to
take her husband to a cancer center,
but their general-practice doctor said
he would never treat him again if he
went elsewhere. (This person did go to
a center, has recovered and is not worrying about the doctor not treating
him again.)*

*An eighty-two-year-old individual
whose surgeon wanted to do immediate lung surgery from a spot seen on an
X ray. This patient had no previous
X ray to compare or any consultation
with an oncologist or any other doctor.
(He went to a cancer center, where he
was told he did not have cancer and
that surgery was totally unnecessary.
The spot was a result of childhood tuberculosis.)*

*An individual whose surgeon said
immediate lung surgery was necessary
because of an X ray spot. There was no*

second opinion. The surgery was per-
formed and was found to be totally un-
necessary. The patient still had to go
through the months of recuperation
and expense.

A well-known celebrity whose lung
had been removed. The surgeon said
he needed chemotherapy; the family
doctor said he knew that the cancer was
totally removed and that there was no
need to go through the discomfort of
chemotherapy. (I visited him eight
months later, after he had chosen the
easy way. The cancer had metastasized
in the other lung with no possible
treatment. He died two days later.)

I could go on and on from the thousands of
phone calls I have received. To me, they
proved the obvious need for this type of program in every city in this country. Not only is
it a tremendous psychological benefit to the
patient and his friends and relatives, but it has
been a factor in actually saving many lives.

Supposedly, one of the most deadly cancers
is that of the pancreas. We have several volunteers who have been cured of pancreas cancer.

I was talking to an oncologist who listed three serious types of cancer. I asked him why he left out pancreas. His reply was he wouldn't mind having pancreas cancer today, because he thought he could beat it. A statement like this to a newly diagnosed pancreas-cancer patient can not only make the difference between life and death but can dramatically improve the quality of life.

The Cancer Hot Line is totally free in Kansas City. Any services or products needed must be donated. Everything is done by volunteers. We do not accept contributions, and when offered, we suggest they be made to a church or a hospital. In other cities, contributions may be accepted.

From its inception in 1980, the Cancer Hot Line has received calls from over 30,000 cancer patients or related parties. This does not include the many unrecorded calls for information. We have more than 150 wonderful volunteers who are willing and ready to give of their personal time with the sole reward being the satisfaction in having helped other human beings.

chapter 11

Establishing the treatment panel

 On that same flight home from Houston after being told that I was cured, I tried to figure out what avenues, in addition to the Hot Line, I could pursue. Thinking back again to my personal experiences, I realized that I was here and alive because I went to Houston. If I had stayed in Kansas City and listened to the original doctor, I might not be alive today.

Many people, because of time, money or poor advice, are unable to go to a major cancer center. These individuals are entitled to a chance at life. The resources are available in every major town. All it would take is the proper structuring of these resources. This thinking would eventually lead to the establishment of the second part of my project—the Cancer Treatment Panel.

I discussed these ideas in their embryonic

stage with an acquaintance. She had had cancer and had completed some six years of chemo-therapy. She arranged a luncheon with a top surgical oncologist.

He listened to my idea that the average Kansas City resident should be able to get the best advice for the treatment of cancer without having to leave the city. He liked the idea of a group of oncologists to prescribe treatment. He was in the process of building a new building next to a hospital for his own cancer clinic. He wanted to house this panel in his building. Furthermore, he said that oncologists would be happy to donate their time without charge and serve on a panel like this to help others. If I would agree to house this panel in his clinic, he said, he would get the doctors to staff the panel.

This surprised me for many reasons. First, I did not think the first person I talked to would be so enthusiastic about my idea. Second, I had no thought that doctors would donate their services. This, in itself, meant that great things were possible.

I explained to the surgeon that one of the fundamental requirements for the panel to be successful was to meet in a neutral place. This was necessary so that doctors could refer their patients without fear of losing them. For the patient to walk through a door with an oncologist's name on it, or for the panel to meet in the same hospital each time, would keep doctors from referring their patients. Even though the luncheon ended without anything tangible accomplished, I felt good about the prospects. I decided to arrange to have lunch every day with someone who could help to establish these cancer programs.

At a noon meeting with an oncologist at a major teaching hospital, I told my story. His response was, "When your doctor told you that you were malignant, he of course arranged for you to come before the tumor board that we used to have." I said, "What tumor board?" He said the hospital had had the finest tumor board in the Midwest until the government recently took away the funding.

After relating my story to the head of a medical society, his response was that it was fortunate the biopsy had been done in the right hospital; he assumed that the doctor had immediately taken my case to the tumor board. Again my response was, "What tumor board?"

This made me realize two very important basic facts: Many doctors will not voluntarily recommend a patient elsewhere, and, as with the Cancer Hot Line, publicity would be the key to the success of this program.

Most cancers are diagnosed by doctors other than oncologists. They are diagnosed by family doctors, gynecologists, ear-nose-and-throat doctors, and so on. Some of these doctors do not want to take the chance of losing revenue, do not want to take the chance of having their patient believe some other doctor is more knowledgeable than they are, do not want to fool around with the inconvenience of a consultant, or honestly believe that they know everything there is to know about cancer. The patients of these doctors probably are most in need of the second opinion. Therefore, we must get the patient to demand the second opinion, since we can't always rely on the doctor to recommend it. The way to do this is through publicity.

At lunch with another medical oncologist, I asked how often he treated a patient for cancer without a second opinion. This man, in his sixties, replied that he had never in his career treated a cancer patient without a second opinion. Furthermore, he always insisted on a second opinion from someone other than an associate of his. This was for four reasons:

• Cancer is a very serious disease that grows geometrically. If it is not treated properly the first time, there is often no second chance.

• He is human and could make a mistake.

• Someone else could see something that he doesn't see.

• Someone else could know something that he doesn't know.

I thought this was a profound statement. I wished that every doctor treating a cancer patient could hear this. My conclusion from this statement is that any doctor treating a cancer patient without a second opinion is not practicing medicine, but trying to play God. I thought it was only God who was supposed to be perfect, know everything and never make a mistake.

Another doctor told me about a sizable clinic in a small town in Missouri that treats people from a wide area. It has no scanner with which to give a bone, brain or liver scan, vital to the determination of the extent of many cancers. Yet, this clinic diagnoses, treats and buries many cancer cases.

From all this information and other conversations too numerous to mention, the plans for the Cancer Treatment Panel were formalized. I decided to have the first panel meet on September 2, 1980. My wife and I invited forty-four top oncologists and other doctors directly working against cancer to our home one evening for cocktails. Thirty-five of these doctors and their spouses accepted our invitation. I felt that this was a good turnout.

After I presented the plans, hopes and dreams of this Cancer Treatment Panel, their reaction was elicited. One surgeon felt that it was ridiculous that I insisted on no fees, because doctors had to get paid. One medical doctor was opposed to it, because he had no time to become involved in it, and he was opposed to anything in which he could not become personally involved. A third doctor thought we should do it by closed-circuit TV.

The important thing is that thirty-two doctors were in favor of it. Our dream was fast becoming a reality. My wife and I sat up talking for hours that night relishing the enthusiastic support of the group. The Cancer Treatment Panel had become a reality.

The Cancer Treatment Panel was composed

of five doctors meeting regularly in a neutral setting—a medical oncologist, a surgeon, a radiologist, a pathologist and a psychiatrist or psychologist. In Kansas City, they met at 5 P.M. Tuesdays at a different centrally located hospital each time. The doctors worked on a rotating basis. From time to time, doctors specializing in other fields were invited to sit in. Up to four patients a week were seen. These patients were required to bring all their records, including X rays, slides and medical reports.

Technically, they were being referred to the panel by their doctor, by his giving them their records for presentation there. The purpose of the panel was to review the doctor's proposed treatment and approve it or recommend additions or alternatives. The recommendations of the panel, in addition to being fully discussed in front of the patient, were written down and sent to the referring doctor, with a copy for the patient.

This idea of holding all discussions openly and frankly in front of the patient and any relatives or friends he cares to bring is unique in the medical world. Furthermore, the psychiatrist or psychologist proved to be a key mem-

ber of the panel. Not only did a majority of
patients leave with a recommended improved
medical treatment, but every patient left with
an improved state of mind. They all felt better
and had more confidence about what was
ahead of them.

Two volunteers from a mental-health
association would sit in the waiting room
with patients and their family and friends
until they got to see the panel. Often these
volunteers called the patients after their
session with the panel to see if they could be
of further assistance.

One of the reasons for family or friends
being present is that the patient, being so
deeply involved, may tend not to hear things
as they are said. Later on, the people in at-
tendance can present their interpretation of
what was said. Furthermore, we know that the
cure of cancer requires the support of family
and friends.

After one of the first sessions of the panel,
I wrote the following fundamental principles
to guide future panels. Doctors at first had
reservations about them but, after trying
them, came to adopt them with respect and
admiration.

- Every patient is to leave happy for having been heard by the panel.
- The patient appears in front of the panel with his or her spouse and relatives and friends.
- All discussions of treatment are held by doctors openly in front of the patient.
- Recommendations are put in writing and sent to the patient's doctor, with a copy for the patient.
- Since there is always hope in psychology or prayer, no patient is ever denied hope.

In the first two sessions, in my lay opinion, the lives of two patients were saved. Both were being treated but were given no hope for recovery. After a lengthy review of each case and a considerable amount of discussion, the doctors on these panels recommended additional forms of therapy and felt that the patient had an excellent chance of being cured. The panel reemphasized the need and importance of a prompt and qualified second opinion in cancer cases as well as the importance of psychological support.

The panel planned to meet in the evening before Christmas Eve with only one patient scheduled to appear. We called the doctor who

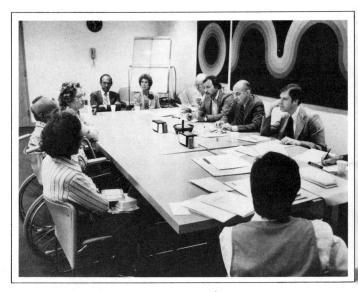

A cancer treatment panel in progress

was leading the panel and asked if he wanted to postpone this patient a week. His reply was that if this man felt it was worth it for him to come before the panel the evening before Christmas Eve, then the panel would be there. And so they were. I understand that the panel proved to be beneficial for this individual. This proves to me the dedication of these wonderful doctors.

An internist told me, "As a general practitioner, I diagnose many cancer cases. Even though I don't know the latest and best treatments for many types of cancer, I must prescribe treatment, because if I send the patient to an oncologist, he'll probably get chemotherapy; if I send the patient to a surgeon, he'll probably get surgery; if I send the patient to a radiotherapist, he'll probably get radiation therapy. I have to decide the treatment for the patient, even though I'm not an expert. Now, I can send them to your panel, where they appear in front of all the disciplines, and they get the right treatment prescribed the first time."

My goals:

• Urge every doctor not to play God. See that every cancer patient receives a qualified, independent second opinion.

• Encourage every cancer patient to find a doctor and a treatment in which he can have confidence and that he will follow all the way through.

• Encourage every cancer patient to play it on the safe side, the conservative side. Often there is no second chance.

• Encourage every cancer patient to use a positive mental attitude to think away the cancer. Remember, even if no one can prove it will help, it can't hurt. If it does nothing but keep your mind off the alternative, that's something.

• Encourage every cancer patient to be selfish. Think of yourself first and do just what you feel like doing. Talk about it openly if you feel like it. It will help to discuss your thoughts with loved ones and friends. Don't be considerate of a doctor who says you won't make it. Change and find one who says he will try to cure you.

• Encourage every cancer patient not to turn away from his loved ones and friends. You have nothing contagious. You need companionship, and maybe with their help and prayers you can stick around for many years and be with them.

chapter 12

Organizing the Cancer Management Center

In the year and a half of its exis-
tance, the Cancer Treatment
Panel saw approximately 250
patients. A great deal of knowledge was gained. Among other
things, the doctors felt that they should have
an opportunity to examine the patient's records prior to the panel. They possibly should
have a chance to research the particular type of
cancer in advance. They wanted an opportunity to discuss the case amongst themselves
prior to discussing the case openly in front of
the patient and their family and friends. They
conscientiously felt that they were depriving
the patients of the best possible solutions.

Annette and I have a goal of giving the next
person who gets cancer the best possible chance
of beating it. We do not want to be associated
with anything that is second-best. If the

doctors had this many objections to what was agreed to be the best thing available, then we had to find a way to improve it.

In keeping with the thought that people who have cancer and do not have the time or money to go out of town should still have the opportunity to receive proper treatment, we decided to try to open a treatment center to serve them. We would incorporate the best aspects of all the centers around the country. We could probably get the primary structure built for around $100 million. That, however, was not a realistic approach.

Furthermore, all the resources were currently available in Kansas City, but they were fragmented. We have radiation-therapy equipment sufficient for any need scattered throughout the various hospitals. As a matter of fact, a recent survey showed that we had a surplus of radiation equipment. We have a sufficient quantity of oncologists, pathologists, radiation therapists, radiologists, surgeons, hematologists and other specialists who, we believe, are as qualified as any in the country. We certainly have enough hospital beds and related facilities. The problem is, as in most cities, that all of this is fragmented.

We spent many hours discussing the problem and trying to figure out a practical solution. How could we as laymen organize the available resources and do this so it could be copied in other cities?

The critical element in successfully treating cancer is in promptly receiving the proper treatment. In other words, it is doctors and knowledge that successfully treat cancer, not brick and mortar. We know that cancer is more than a hundred different diseases. There is no relationship between breast cancer and brain cancer other than the name and the fact that they are both rapidly dividing cells. It is impossible for one general doctor to be informed on the latest and best treatment for every type of cancer. Furthermore, it is impossible for one specialist, such as a surgeon, radiotherapist or oncologist, to know the very latest and best treatment in his own specialty for every one of the more than one hundred different types of cancer.

Our initial thoughts were subsequently substantiated in the draft of the May, 1985 publication of the National Institutes of Health entitled *Cancer Control Objectives for the Nation 1985-2000*. It states, "The application of the state of the art treatment is complex. At all levels of the health service delivery system—from the primary care physician who has initial contact with the patient to specialists directing the cancer treatment—physician knowledge is not yet optimal. That knowledge should include an appreciation for state-of-the-art treatment information and an interest in ensuring early multidisciplinary decision making….For about 70 percent of cancers, optimal therapy derives from multidisciplinary discussions. The relative rarity of some of the most responsive tumors means that proficient treatment can be maintained only at some major cancer centers. …Malpractice considerations may result in physicians selecting "safe" therapy, which neither offers significant risk nor the chance of cure….A major determinant of outcome for most newly diagnosed cancer patients with curable disease hinges on early multi-disciplinary treatment planning and the availability of expertise and resources to carry out such a treatment plan."

On this premise, we came to the conclusion that our goal was the establishment of panels similar to the Cancer Treatment Panel. Furthermore, this series of panels should have a home in an absolutely neutral site. We determined that the ideal site would be on an academic campus with no medical facilities at hand. In our case, this is the University of Missouri at Kansas City.

Now, how do we go about getting all the doctors and hospitals to cooperate and make it a joint effort? We would make it a not-for-profit organization to be governed by a board of directors composed of one representative from each major hospital in the metropolitan area. To our knowledge, this is the only time all the hospitals in the area have cooperated on any project.

Four outstanding physicians representing different specialties met at our home from November 1981 through April 1982 to plan the details. All the planning was based on a set of fundamental principles that were derived from one primary statement, "Everything will be done that is for the best interest of the patient, and nothing will be done that is not for the best interest of the patient."

Because there is a great deal of psychology involved in the recovery from cancer, it was felt that the Center needed to be in a prestigious-appearing facility. While the University of Missouri at Kansas City (UMKC) was an ideal setting for our needs, we would prove to be a tremendous asset to the University, which is involved in research and dissemination of knowledge. Our Center would be a focal point for cancer activities in the area and eventually be part of a network comprising several universities, which would share knowledge and progress made in cancer care.

It was agreed that our goal was to help cancer patients, not build a mammoth institution. Our hopes were for this Center to be a prototype to be copied by other institutions of learning around the country. The Center was designed with three examining rooms and one conference room.

The University provided a ground-floor area of a very imposing stone building on the campus with a private entrance and handsome exterior sign. Our decorator, James Gohl, donated his services in designing and decorating the Center, and he did an outstanding job.

The discussion as to the name of the Center was interesting, and it indicates the uniqueness of this disease called *cancer.* This is not a diagnostic center. Patients who come here have already been diagnosed as having cancer. This is not a treatment center. We do not have an IV bottle, an X-ray machine, or anything else to give any kind of treatment. A physician can send his patient here with no fear that he will lose the patient to the Center. What we are is strictly a management center to recommend the proper treatment for cancer. Think about this! Have you ever heard of any other disease that requires management?

To assure our continuous personal support of this unique concept, we lent our personal names, Richard and Annette Bloch, and called it the R. A. Bloch Cancer Management Center.

On May 1, 1982, the R. A. Bloch Cancer Management Center became a reality. The date chosen was most significant and meaningful to us; it marked the second anniversary of the day I was told I was cured. It also was another step in fulfilling my promise to devote my life to helping people with cancer. Here is a project accomplished not only without any government money, but also with relatively little private money.

There is no charge to anyone to attend the panel. There is no bank account. No donations are accepted. The doctors generally will not even treat a patient they see on the panel. They want this to be truly an independent second opinion. They are donating their time to see that the patient has the best chance of beating cancer as easily as possible.

Volunteers organized a program to assist patients coming from outside the city. These volunteers are available to discuss and help with housing, transportation, restaurants, and so forth. We know what a traumatic experience it is to go away from home for medical treatment. We want to make this as simple and pleasant as possible.

A great deal of discussion was held as to which geographical areas we should accept patients from. The initial purpose of the Center was to help people in Kansas City. However, if a person cannot get proper service wherever they are, we should be available.

Initially, we received a tremendous amount of publicity from the Associated Press, United Press International, and various radio and TV networks. On the morning the Center opened, I was there with the Acting Director and the Director of Admissions. The three of us handled over two hundred calls from people all over the country wanting to come to the Center. The response was extremely gratifying, but, at the same time, it presented three major problems. People who were already receiving qualified care in their community wanted to come; people thought we had magic solutions, and there was no way we could handle this volume. Cancer cases must be treated promptly, and there was no way we could see so many people right away.

Our board of directors promptly made two restrictions: first, no more publicity on such a grand scale for the time being; and second, admissions were restricted to Missouri and Kansas. Why have someone travel hundreds of miles when a major cancer center is nearby? For individuals residing outside of Missouri or Kansas, institutions that have stated they will, if specifically requested, make available a multi-disciplinary second opinion with the patient and friends or family present are listed on page 167.

Much discussion was also held about the concept of physician referral—that is, whether to require a patient's physician to call before the patient could be admitted. Most physicians would prefer doctor referral, so we started off requiring it.

An individual called me and said that his doctor refused to refer his father. The doctor's refusal was based on the fact that he knew the patient would be dead in two years, so there was no point in wasting the patient's time or the Center's time. When our doctors heard this, they promptly took in the patient. I understand the patient left with a more optimistic outlook. Presently, the Center would like a doctor's referral or the opportunity to talk with the doctor as to the reason for his refusal to refer.

The Center does not want a patient who runs from doctor to doctor for no good reason. For the patient who is not satisfied with his doctor's prognosis or has any doubt in his mind about his doctor and cannot find qualified help locally, this Center or any more convenient Center should be available. Remember, you have to be selfish with your disease!

Of the first group of patients, all but one had to request their respective doctors to refer them. One patient whose doctor opposed his coming was found not to have cancer at all, even though this doctor was treating him for it.

The last few paragraphs may give the impression that many doctors are not in favor of the Cancer Management Center. The good doctors, the quality doctors, the qualified doctors are solidly in favor of the Cancer Management Center. These are the doctors who would normally insist that their patients get an independent second opinion prior to treatment. We have over one hundred physicians, from all specialties and representing all institutions in the area; they not only are in favor of the concept, but have volunteered to serve on the panels and have been approved by a rigorous screening committee.

The panel makes a point to never shake the patient's faith in their physician. These wonderful doctors generally concur with the patient's current or recommended treatments. This reinforces their confidence and enables them to partake of their treatments with more certainty. Occasionally the doctors will recommend investigating additional methods of therapy or different treatments. This can only increase the patient's chance for success. The patient always leaves knowing they are better-off for having come to the panel.

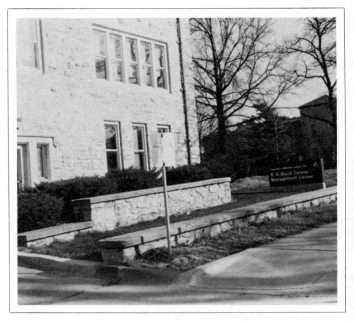

R.A. Bloch Cancer Management Center

At the front entrance of the R. A. Bloch Cancer Management Center is a slogan for all physicians and patients to read and practice:

> To achieve excellence
> Attempt perfection
> Less is unacceptable.

chapter 13

A look at
the future

We have done a great deal of writing about my personal case and about cancer treatment as it exists today. Let's go a little further and explore what the future may hold. Realizing that most people reading this book have cancer or have a friend or relative with cancer today, why talk about the future? Because the future is not five or ten years from now. The future is this afternoon, tomorrow or the next day. By the time this book is printed and you have read it, a great deal of the future will already be here.

The National Cancer Institute is spending over $1^1/_2$ billion dollars a year to eliminate the cause and create a cure for cancer. It has been in existence more than eighteen years. Tremendous strides have been made in treatment in this period. Yet, recent statistics show only 49 percent of serious cases survive five years or are technically cured.

M. D. Anderson is an institution to which many physicians will refer their patients only after they believe there is no more hope. Supposedly, they get the worst of the cases and often after a physician has experimented with various treatments. An official of M. D. Anderson told me their cure rate was 52 percent when the national statistic was 42 percent. I asked what he believes their cure rate would be if they received patients promptly upon diagnosis. His answer was, "Conservatively 62 percent."

What does this mean? This means that, on an average, if patients with all serious cancers were treated promptly, properly and thoroughly, better than one out of three who now will die, would be cured.

How do we disseminate this currently existing knowledge and ability to save lives to the patients who need it? The billions of dollars invested and the millions of lives lost and hours spent to establish these life saving treatments are totally wasted if one doctor treating one patient is unaware that these treatments are available.

A company called CompuServe in Columbus, Ohio, has gigantic computers and a private telephone network to most cities in America. H&R Block acquired this company. Certain major newspapers use computers to set their paper. These computers feed directly into our giant computer. I have a $299 Radio Shack terminal in my home that I connect to my phone and my television set, and I can read any part of any paper I choose. I spent many sleepless nights going over in my mind how I could apply this remarkable technology toward the goals I so desperately want to achieve. Annette and I would sit and talk for hours knowing that somewhere, somehow there was a way. We believed the R. A. Bloch Cancer Management Center would bring the best possible treatment to Kansas City and other major cities who would eventually copy it. But what about all the people living in small towns and rural areas where there is a lack of qualified cancer physicians?

We came up finally with a concept that we feel is unique and exciting. It is to put every known therapy for every type of cancer under every condition into a computer. A doctor anywhere in America, on his own or his hospital's computer terminal, can make a local telephone call and be connected with our main frame in Columbus, Ohio. He would enter the type of cancer, location, age, sex, and present medical problems. The computer would immediately come back with the recommended treatments from the different Centers, along with necessary precautions because of current physical conditions. In the 12 percent of cases that would require experimental therapy, the computer would not describe the treatment but would show where the relevant experimental therapy was being offered. Furthermore, for a subsequent period of one year, the computer would automatically call the physician back to advise of any changes or improvements in the treatments.

To get all this information into a computer is a monumental task. We know of no way of doing this other than through the National Cancer Institute. If the premise is right, that prompt, proper and thorough treatment could increase survival from 42 percent to 62 percent, if more than 800,000 Americans get cancer each year, then this program could conceivably save 160,000 lives each year. The results would make the enormous investment well worth while.

A total cost of this service, including the long-distance charge, computer time and call backs, would be a flat ten dollars. We intend to promote this service by saying that anyone who believes that his or her life is worth ten dollars will ask his doctor to get this for him and will read it and discuss it along with his doctor. He will then know all the options and be able to be involved in the treatment, one of the requirements for recovery from cancer.

Any doctor hesitant about getting this computer printout would be implying that he knows more than all the scientists and doctors across the nation in treating this particular kind of cancer.

In November 1981, Annette and I made an appointment with Dr. DeVita, director of the National Cancer Institute in Bethesda, Maryland, to discuss this concept. His reaction to this idea was extremely favorable, and his comment was that it was the greatest idea to reduce the mortality from cancer that he had heard since he had been practicing medicine. He assured us that it would get done.

As this program holds tremendous potential, we feared our aim could be misconstrued by certain persons suggesting we were doing

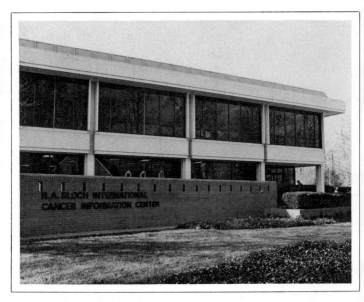

R.A. Bloch International Cancer Information Center,
home of Protocol Data Query (PDQ),
in Bethesda, Maryland

this to give CompuServe, a subsidiary of
H&R Block, business. Annette and I therefore sold our holdings in H&R Block, Inc., in
November 1982, and I resigned from the
board of directors to confirm our sincere belief
in this program.

PDQ has been available since 1984. I suggest patients call 1-800-4-Cancer and request
the state-of-the-art therapy for their specific
type and stage of cancer only. Also, they
should request all current open protocols from
everywhere in the United States for their specific type and stage of cancer. This will give
you peace of mind knowing your doctor is giving you the best possible treatment. If you
have any questions, ask your doctor.

———————

To continue on the theory of prompt,
proper and thorough treatment with a positive
mental attitude, let's discuss the mental-atti-
tude part. Several things have happened lately
to make me all the more aware of how important mental attitude is in recovery.

So that you won't get the wrong impression, I want to emphatically state that it takes

six factors to recover from cancer: first is the finest possible medical treatment; second is the finest possible medical treatment; third, fourth and fifth are the finest possible medical treatment; and sixth is a positive mental attitude! Without all six, the cancer patient will not make it.

In the early stages of our Cancer Hot Line, we had two "cured" volunteers who had to stop taking phone calls because they could not bear to talk about cancer-related problems. I told Annette at the time that in spite of what their doctors had told them, they were not through with cancer. Since that time, one has passed away and the other has a new malignancy. I sensed that they subconsciously felt that they were destined to die of cancer. Sometimes when one feels strongly enough about something, it can almost be willed to happen.

In visiting the Cancer Management Center with a New York physician who is interested in duplicating it, we met a patient who refused to allow her friends to know that she had cancer. He agreed that she had condemned herself to death if she could not bring about a change in her mental attitude.

I met a very cheerful lady who has had three

bouts with cancer. She said that her attitude is very positive and she is going to beat it this time too. She has a wonderful doctor. I asked whether her doctor gave her a favorable prognosis. She said she had never asked him, because she was afraid of what he would say. This meant to me that way down deep she did not truly believe she would make it; otherwise she would want to hear what the doctor, in whom she had faith, would say. She needed some psychological support.

Realizing the importance of mental attitude in the recovery from cancer, we have put together a panel of two psychologists, a psychiatrist and a social worker. Their goal is to design a simple, short questionnaire that can be graded precisely. This would show a cancer patient that psychological assistance could conceivably improve the receptiveness to successful medical treatment.

With the help of a group of phychologists and phychiatrists from the National Cancer Institute and another group from Memorial Sloan-Kettering, this quiz has been developed. It is available in the book *Fighting Cancer*, or can be obtained without charge by sending a self-addressed stamped envelope

to Quiz, Cancer Connection, 4410 Main
Street, Kansas City, MO 64111.

At each meeting of the National Cancer
Advisory Board, we are apprised of the dramatic progress in cancer knowledge and treatments. It is coming so rapidly that it is
mind-boggling.

The greatest progress being made today is
with monoclonal antibodies that are not only
used for early detection and staging but armed
with various substances for actual treatment
and immunotherapy. This would include in-
terlukens, interfuron and tumor necrosis factors, each attempting to strengthen the
immune system to avoid or cure cancer without toxicity.

We were told that changes in this area are
coming about so rapidly that research projects
started six months ago are obsolete today. Of
course, the greatest hope of all is to some day
have an injection that will make a person immune to cancer.

What I am trying to emphasize is that even
if there is no cure known today for a particular
type of cancer, the individual should make
every effort to fight the disease, because
tomorrow a successful treatment could be

discovered.

Annette and I receive many letters from individuals thanking us for giving them courage or pointing them in the right direction to try to fight their cancer. We appreciate and treasure each of these letters. Each one of them makes all our efforts worthwhile. Normally, we do not share these with anyone; however, we want to make one exception with the following letter because it demonstrates so vividly two specific factors. First is the type of individual we strive hardest to help: that is the one who honestly and sincerely wants to help themself; the one who will pull out all the stops and keep trying, no matter how many road blocks are encountered.

Second is to answer our most common critic: the one who accuses us of giving false hope. After all, I was told I was going to die. There was no hope. And here I am. How much worse off is this lady for having hope? You tell me! (All names have been changed.)

On the front of the note paper is printed, "Life is a miracle, and the right to live is a gift. It's wrapped in a ribbon woven with dreams, and whether you are very young or very old, life is filled with wonder and surprises."

July 19, 1985

Dear Dick-

*I'm sorry to be so long in letting you
know what happened to me. You were so
kind and patient and helpful. Seems I
called you so many times. In Sarasota,
lovely as it is, one is cut off from the real
world' - where research is being done. It's
'status quo' here. Had I not been led to
where I am, I would have been left to die
here of melanoma. But I was not because of
the Hot Line, the Cancer Information Service in Bethesda and a girl (because my oncologist refused to avail herself of your
PDQ) (Ed. Note: The Cancer Information
Service had told the patient on the phone
that they had enough currently active protocols for her type of cancer 'to fill a Manhat-
tan telephone directory. Her physician said
she did not have time to read them, that
none of them could help her and she would
die anyway). The girl [I spoke to at the
Cancer Information Service] gave me ran-
dom places on the East coast and in the
South were PDQ showed research being
done. Some of the programs are 'down'*

however.

She told me, as you did, about Dr. White at the University of Miami. His program for melanoma is down but after 3 calls to him, he referred us (and made an advance call) to Dr. Black at Mt. Sinai in Miami Beach. Dr. Black is chief of general surgery and oncology. He was chief of staff till 2 years ago at Barnes in St. Louis. He's been researching melanoma 13 years (he is only 40 now!). He is working with Duke and Emery on immunization therapy.

Jack, my husband, sat in my oncologist's office 3 hours to make her call Dr. Black. You see, Dr. Black called my Jack after Dr. White called him but could not make an appointment to see me until the oncologist called him. Jack sat right there till she finally called. She told him I'd had a node out before that and scans showed another close by. Otherwise no invasion of vital organs and blood count normal.

We made an appointment and saw him the next week. He examined and talked to us at length. He told me he had a program funded by NCI for 40 melanoma patients and if he took me, I'd be the 37th. But first he made an appointment for a few days later for an all day session in nuclear medicine - 9:30 AM til 4:30 PM - then pre-op work-up (i.e. X rays, EKG, etc.) for surgery of large node and the whole field of nodes in left neck area (modified radical). This all happened a week ago today.

One of country's top head and neck men did the surgery, Black assisting. Path report: Large node seen on scan malignant and all others removed were 'clean'. I look rather like I'd had a head transplant. Tomorrow we will be in Miami again for staple and stitch removal and then back next Thursday to begin 'the program' - I'm in-praise God.

The program consists of 1 shot every week for 13 weeks and then every other week for a year. Because I live so far away, Dr. Black will allow a doctor here to administer the serum (whatever it is) and I'll only have to go to Miami every 3 months. Isn't that lovely.

Best part? I was admitted as a 'teaching patient' as I explained our financial situation and have no insurance at this time. No cost for anything. Isn't God wonderful? We've had rotten luck so long. I adore them over at Mt. Sinai...As the doctor who did

*my surgery said, 'Sue, don't look at the sta-
tistics. You're a human being and your attitude is great.'*

*I called to thank Rabbi Gold for insisting
Jack and I come hear you the night prior to
our marriage - for if I had not heard you,
taken your pamphlet and finally 20 months
later called you, I would be sentenced to
die.*

*I thank you and Annette who have done
so much good for so many of us about to
give up. Your book was waiting when I got
home and what perfect timing! Thank you
so very much. I was with CBS 15 years - in-
terview shows, news, a syndicated show...if
you ever get too bogged down with speak-
ing engagements please accept my offer of
using me at no charge to speak wherever the
need is. I wish to devote my life to getting
the Hot Line in people's hands and stressing
how one must have more than one person's
opinion.*

*My love and heartfelt thanks to you and
your team...You probably (with God) have
given me extra time here on earth to love
and be loved. God bless you and yours.*

Sue

chapter 14

Summary and conclusions

 Out of everything bad comes something good. Don't misconstrue this statement. I would never choose to have cancer; however, now that it is behind me, I can say that my life is of better quality because of it.

My wife and I had, at the time my cancer was diagnosed, what we thought was a wonderful marriage of thirty-one years. Now it is even better and more fulfilling, because of the experiences we shared, the times we thought our days together were limited, the realization that we can never take each other physically or spiritually for granted, and the idea that we are together sharing our common goal of working to help the next person afflicted with cancer.

My relationship with each of my three daughters and my sons-in-law is more meaningful. Possibly it is because they were given

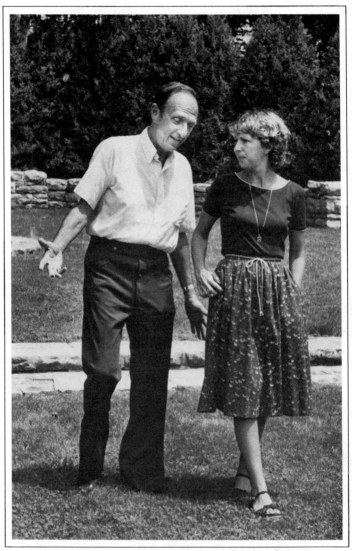

Richard walks in the backyard with his daughter, Nancy Jacob

an opportunity to show and prove their devotion and caring that we mutually treasure every moment together. Our Sunday evening family dinners were routine and enjoyable. Now they are an occasion with a lot more meaning and gratitude for being together. The weekly pool games with my sons-in-law and my brother Leon are now missed only for the most compelling of reasons.

Every day is lived to the fullest. I appreciate everything, and I no longer take one single thing for granted. Maybe my senses have become more acute. The simple pleasure of enjoying a good steak is an event, as is the thrill of seeing the leaves change color in the fall, holding and being with each of my grandchildren, ordering a new car, or watching a good mystery on television. Life is good.

So what conclusions can I reach from my experiences that can be applicable and helpful to you? First, don't feel that, because cancer is so prevalent, it is going to attack you. While statistics say that one out of every four Americans will get cancer, you are not a statistic, you are a person. If you even give a thought to cancer, remember, more people don't get cancer than do, and if you are one of the relatively few people who do, your chances of beating it or controlling it are good. Because of constant advances in medicine, your odds are even better at the time you read this than they were when I wrote it.

According to Dr. Vincent T. DeVita, Jr., Director of the National Cancer Institute, there were fewer than one hundred oncologists in the United States in 1970. Today there are in excess of 3,000. This gives an indication of how rapidly advances in the treatment of cancer are being made.

Some people believe that cancer is caused by the mind. We know statistically that when a traumatic event, such as the loss of a loved one, retirement, business failure, et cetera, occurs, the incidence of cancer rises dramatically. Logically it is, therefore, safe to assume that worrying about cancer could be a factor in bringing it on. That is not to say it would, just that it possibly could.

I believe that getting cancer is not a simple, single action. My father smoked until he died at age ninety-five, and he did not have cancer. On the other hand, I smoked and did get lung cancer. Therefore, I personally believe that it takes a combination of two things to produce cancer: it takes the carcinogen, or cancer-causing agent, such as cigarettes, along with the trauma.

Therefore, having never been afflicted with cancer, if you could possibly control your thought processes, you could be helping yourself to avoid getting cancer.

In the past year, I have noticed through phone calls and patients appearing before our Panel that more tumors were discovered through routine physical examinations or self-examinations than any other source. I cannot stress strongly enough the importance of having regular checkups and following any advice that your physician may give you about self-examination.

If you feel an ache or a pain or notice a lump, don't assume that you have cancer. See your doctor promptly, explain your fears, and take his word if it is not cancer. Pin down what it is, what the treatment is and how long before it will be better. If things proceed as he indicated, your mind should be at ease. My being misdiagnosed by two doctors is more the exception than the rule, so don't panic about doctors.

Never compare your symptoms with those of anyone else; you are an individual and only your doctor can properly tell you what your symptoms mean. I have had people call telling me that they had the same exact pain in their shoulder and arm as I did. So, they are sure that they have the same type of cancer that I did, even though their doctors assure them they do not. As it was pointed out earlier, every case of cancer, like a fingerprint, is unique.

Once a doctor has told you that it is malignant or may be malignant, make up your mind right then and there that you are going to do everything within your power to beat it. The first thing this means is to never look back. Don't ever ask, "Why didn't the doctor discover this before?" or "Why didn't I do something last month when I first noticed it?" or "Why did my spouse allow me to smoke?" or, or, or—. Every individual has a limited amount of energy. Don't waste any of it looking back. Rather, direct this valuable energy into positive action of prompt, proper and thorough treatment. Do everything possible from this moment on, so that you will never be able to look back and say, "I wish I would have . . ."

If any one factor is critical, it is the need for prompt action. As was said, many people learn of their cancer through a routine physical examination. They are probably feeling fairly healthy. It is so easy to procrastinate when nothing really bothers you. You feel exactly the same as you did an hour before, when you walked into the doctor's office. It is difficult to translate those three little words "it is malignant" into a disease that is potentially lethal.

Cancer will never be as treatable as it is today. At some point in the future, it is probably not treatable. Whether this point is one year from now, one month from now, or tomorrow, nobody knows. At any rate, it can only possibly do damage to postpone treatment. Find the proper doctor to manage your treatment today. If he suggests additional tests, take them as soon as they can be scheduled. When he suggests a specific treatment, start that treatment that day. A day lost here and there could mean the difference between success and failure in treating cancer.

At this point, I would like to urge doctors to consider their obligation to their patients in regard to complete truthfulness when telling the patient that he has cancer. I will never fault a doctor for being totally honest with the

patient. I will always disagree with the rare
doctor who confuses honesty with a desire to
play God. Any doctor who says that it is un-
treatable is in reality saying that he, personally, does not know the proper treatment.
There is no way he could conceivably know
what every cancer center in America, or in the
world, could concurrently be doing with that
type of cancer. I have no objection to a doctor
saying that he, personally, does not know the
proper treatment, or even to his saying that he
has personally never seen anyone beat this particular type. However, he will be glad to refer
the patient to someone more knowledgeable
or make phone calls in connection with this.

Any doctor who tells a patient that he has
three to six months to live or gives him any
time limit is, in fact, trying to play God. If he
wants to impress the patient with his knowledge of statistics, he is welcome to accurately
quote statistics. Along with this he should, in
all honesty, explain to that patient that the patient is not a statistic. Statistics are composed
of large masses of people discovering the disease over a period of time prior to the present
by all possible means, in all possible stages
and taking treatment in all possible ways, in-

cluding failing to take treatments. These statistics can serve only as a guideline; they are not applicable to any individual. For no other reason, an individual's prognosis would vary with his desire to live.

I would like to urge the doctors also to consider the state of mind a patient is in when he breaks the news. It is so important to tell the complete truth but to tell it in a gentle and kind way without destroying hope.

Hope—a very little word with so much meaning behind it! I lived for five days without hope, and I want to go on record as saying that my life, during those five days, was far worse than at any time during the "horrible" ordeal of tests or treatments.

While we are on the subject of hope, let us discuss the idea of hope being partly responsible for the successful treatment of cancer. There are two possibilities. Hope will extend the number of days a person has to live or it will not.

For the sake of discussion, let us assume that hope will not increase the quantity of life. There is no question in anyone's mind that hope will improve the quality of life. If a person has only so many days to live on this earth, there is no question that those days with a better quality are preferable to the same number of days with poor quality. Furthermore, no one could maintain that a better quality of life could possibly *shorten* the number of days. To the contrary, it is not only possible, but probable, that an improved quality of life could and would cause an *improved quantity* of life. Therefore, when a doctor takes hope away from a patient, he is destroying the patient. When a doctor, in all honesty, gives genuine hope, not false hope, to a patient, he is improving the quality of his life, giving him a reason and a desire to fight for his life and probably extending the quantity of time.

On the subject of total honesty, a criticism I have of a few doctors is that they tell their patient what they believe the patient wants to hear rather than the complete truth. For example, a surgeon who says "I got it all out" can honestly only mean he got out what he could see. One million cancer cells, being the size of the head of a pin and floating easily in the bloodstream or the lymph system, could be lodged in parts of the body never investigated by the surgeon.

Also, complete honesty cannot be present

with any doctor who would treat a cancer patient without first completing all possible diagnostic tests available today.

In a memorandum by the National Cancer Institute dated October 23, 1981, entitled "Community Clinic Oncology Program" it states: " . . . less than 12 percent of patients presenting with any given malignant disease problem would be required as protocol entries to meet experimental program needs." This is referring to the selection of patients for whom there is no known standard successful therapy to be used in the "development of research strategies and procedures." Considering this statement further, it would indicate that there is a standard, proven, "successful," known therapy for over 88 percent of all cancers. Since this means there is a proven method of treatment for better than seven out of eight newly diagnosed patients, make every effort to locate the physician whose knowledge includes this proven therapy.

It is very important for an individual to become intimately involved with his treatment. If you break your leg, it will mend itself in so many days. If you catch a cold, it will generally last seven days no matter what medication you take. In the case of cancer, it is so complex, with so many possible combinations of treatments, that there is no way to sit back and expect it to go away by itself. While there are numerous cases of documented spontaneous remission—that is, the tumor disappearing without any ostensible treatment—it is so rare that an individual would be foolish to put all his hope in this when there are other options available. Get involved. Read all there is to read about your particular type of cancer. Ask questions. Understand everything your doctor is planning to do and why. Augment this with psychotherapy, diet, prayer, vitamins, and anything else your doctor says will not harm you. Make it a point to find people who have been successfully treated for the same kind of cancer. Listen to what they say.

Remember, your single goal is to try to beat cancer. Don't worry about anything or anyone. Be selfish. Do not harbor your fears or your thoughts and allow them to fester inside you. Talk openly about your thoughts and feelings to your loved ones and friends. This not only will help you but will help them feel comfortable, needed, and part of your recovery process. The word was *openly,* not incessantly. It's one thing to discuss, unload your pent-up emotions and put others at ease. It is another thing to bore people with unnecessary gory details.

From our Cancer Treatment Panel, we found that probably the greatest single problem in cancer treatment is the failure of communication between doctor and patient. This is not a single-edged knife, but a double-edged sword. It is very easy for the patient to say the doctor never told him, or why didn't the doctor tell him. In this particular situation, I can see the doctor's problem. He does not want to burden the patient with unnecessary details; he does not desire to dwell on possibilities and may assume that the patient already has the knowledge. On the other hand, I have been brought up to believe that there is no such thing as a bad question. There can only be bad answers. If there is anything you want to know about your illness, there can be no reason for you not to ask your doctor. Usually the doctor is only too happy to answer any question with full explanation.

Before seeing your doctor, take a pencil and paper and list every question for which you would like an answer. Write down whatever bothers or troubles you. If his answer is not perfectly clear to you, keep asking until you understand thoroughly. I have yet to meet the doctor who did not prefer it this way. I would not want a doctor treating me who would not or could not answer my questions.

There is a famous quote, "The worst thing we have to fear is fear itself." For cancer, I would change it to, "The worst thing we have to fear is the unknown." When I saw people with red lines all over them or saw the size of the radiation equipment, I was scared to death. After my first treatment, realizing it hurt no more than getting my picture taken, I looked forward to continued treatment. When something worries you, talk to someone who has already been through it or talk to your doctor. Doing this often can save you a great deal of unnecessary apprehension and fear. Worry is like a rocking chair, it keeps you busy but gets you nowhere.

One of the common worries we hear a great deal about is the potential negative side effects or after effects of various treatments. This can be broken down into numerous areas. First is the person who says he will not take radiation therapy, because his grandfather was severely burned. The strides made in treatments over the years make a science today of what was trial and error. The person refusing chemo-therapy because of possible future heart problems does not realize that scientists know exactly how much of a particular drug a person can tolerate without any adverse effects.

Then there is always the story that sells newspapers about the bad effects of one treatment or another. Remember, there are two million Americans walking around today who have been cured of cancer. Maybe those articles talk about a doctor giving a damaging drug for no good reason or for the sake of money. Don't deny yourself a chance to live because of negative publicity or horror stories. Be certain you get a doctor who is capable and interested in successfully treating you.

A middle-aged lady came before the Cancer Treatment Panel with a lymphoma involving her groin and abdomen. After a lengthy review of her case, the Panel told her she could be very adequately treated with an excellent chance of obtaining a good remission by taking a pill a day. They further assured her that this pill would be tolerated as easily as if she had taken an aspirin. She asked if this treatment was called chemotherapy and when answered in the affirmative, she very flatly and defiantly said that under no circumstances would she submit to chemotherapy. She had read a great deal of recent adverse publicity and would not allow her body to be abused by drugs. She had no objection to taking an aspirin or "standard medicines," but chemotherapy—absolutely not.

The doctors patiently reiterated that this pill would most likely not cause her any uncomfortable symptoms, and her only alternative was to allow the lymphoma to progress to a fatal stage. The frustrating thing was the doctors could almost guarantee her complete remission. Just think how many patients would give anything to be given that kind of prognosis. In so many cases cure cannot be discussed, just hoped for, but rarely guaranteed. After a great deal of compassionate pleading, she finally agreed to take the pill and live. It is a shame to think how a carelessly written article could cost a human life. I have hopes that in the future, newspapers will be more conscientious in their selection of articles and check out the authenticity of the connotation as well as the denotation.

While we are on the subject, be certain that the doctor prescribing your treatment is an oncologist. If you want the treatment given by your family doctor or anyone else, that's fine, as long as it is approved by an oncologist—a doctor who has been trained and board certified in the treatment of cancer. Another reason why an oncologist, or any doctor involved in the treatment of cancer, is so important is that you need a doctor who will treat a whole person, not just a disease. There is no point in curing the cancer and killing the patient, nor is there any advantage in treating the cancer more aggressively than needed and doing unnecessary damage.

If your doctor even hints that he does not want a second opinion before treating you for cancer, I would strongly urge you to have nothing to do with him. A dedicated and conscientious cancer doctor will concur with your obtaining a second opinion prior to treatment. The oath of Hippocrates states, in effect, that nothing shall be done that is not in the best interest of the patient. Supposedly, this is the oath that every doctor is sworn to uphold.

You must have complete faith in the doctor you choose to manage the treatment of your cancer. Remember, you should be selfish. This is your life. Don't let anyone else's ethics affect you. Your ethics are to beat cancer, and nothing else matters. To have the best chance of doing this, you must have a good rapport with your doctor, ability to communicate with him and, above all, absolute confidence in him. If any of these factors is missing, find a doctor who satisfies all three of these requirements.

Whatever this doctor recommends, follow through with it all the way, knowing and sincerely believing that it will successfully treat you. He is giving you these treatments, not just for the sake of giving treatments, but for the sake of getting rid of the cancer.

Don't necessarily look for a "cure" for your cancer. It is possible, with our limited knowledge today, that some cancers cannot be cured. Some can be gotten into complete remission, some into partial remission, and some only controlled. I told a sixty-year-old man that if the doctors could control his cancer for another sixty years, he should settle for that. Don't forget that if the control is only temporary, new treatments are constantly being discovered that could be helpful.

There is a bright side to most cancers. From

my understanding, the faster it grows, the easier it is to treat. Most chemotherapy drugs recognize cancer cells only because they are rapidly multiplying.

Just because a cancer has metastasized does not necessarily mean an unfavorable prognosis. Quite often, certain types of cancer are not found until they have metastasized. If the primary tumor can be successfully treated, the metastasis is usually equally treatable. Again, don't compare your situation with anyone else's and don't listen to any one else's horror stories.

Some people misinterpret the possible pain or weak feeling they get from their treatment. They mistakenly believe their cancer is getting worse. It is perfectly normal and desirable to be affected in this way by certain treatments such as surgery, radiation or chemotherapy. After all, these treatments are trying to kill those weak little cancer cells. The fact that you are always tired or your taste buds have become distorted or certain odors are offensive would more likely indicate that the treatments are working and doing what they are supposed to do.

During your treatment, keep yourself as busy and active as you feel able to, and as your doctor will permit. We had one lady in front of our panel who asked if it was all right for her to continue singing with her church choir. A gentleman wanted to know whether he could continue going to work during chemotherapy. In both cases, the doctors urged these people to engage in all normal activities that they felt physically able to do. If, for the day or two immediately following chemotherapy, they felt weak, it was important to give in and not push. However, after that brief period passed, it was equally important to make yourself live a normal active life.

Don't get impatient, and don't worry "what if?" Communicate with your doctor to get a time frame and thoroughly understand the expected series of feelings and results. Relax and give the treatments a chance to work. If you expect to be on a particular therapy for three months before seeing any results, don't be disappointed to see no results after only thirty days. Know that after the three months there are other options open to you, but do not be concerned about them until you reach that point in time. First things first. Your doctor has selected what he believes is the best and most desirable choice. Have a positive attitude throughout this time, and give this most desirable treatment every chance to work.

Don't look for the easy road, and don't listen to the negatives. Concentrate all your energy into being positive. It isn't always easy, I know, to do this, but it's worth the effort. The easy way—like vitamins, laetril, prayer, and positive attitude, without medical attention—is not always the best way. Your doctor is recommending what he believes is the easiest and best way. If you want to supplement his recommended treatment with anything he says will not harm you or interfere with the treatment, then do it.

If the Lord believed that prayer alone could cure you, then why were so many doctors put on this earth? I am a strong believer in prayer, and I used it constantly during my illness. I believe it should be used in conjunction with proper medical help. Don't forsake any of your options. Use all of them! How lucky we are to be living in a day and age when they are available.

I have learned that when a person thinks he is going to die, he is generally right. To recover takes three conscious decisions:

First, you must decide you want to live. Some people want to die, and cancer is one way out. Make a conscious decision that you

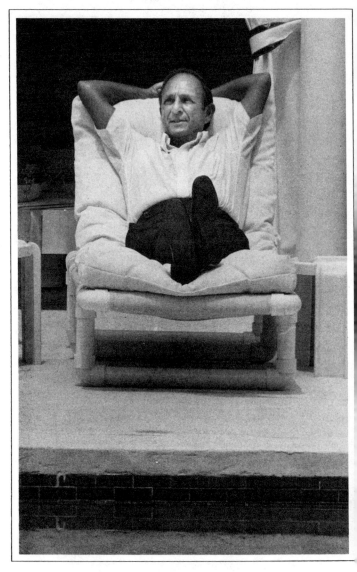

Life for Richard Bloch today is at once far removed yet undeniably tied to his bout with cancer

want to live.

Second, make a conscious decision that you have absolute and complete faith in your doctor and the fact that he will cure you.

Third, make a conscious decision that the treatment he has recommended is the best possible treatment and that it will cure you. Then, and only then, can you have a chance of licking cancer.

Every time Annette and I go to Florida, we go back to that little island in the middle of the New River where we wrote "We Shall Return." Annette, with a stick, draws a heart in the sand and puts in our initials, the date, and writes, "We did return. And we shall continue to return."

Epilogue

My profound appreciation to all the doctors and other volunteers who have so enthusiastically and generously supported and given of themselves to the Cancer Panels and the Cancer Hot Line. The success of these programs would not have been possible without their wholehearted support and dedication.

If the reader has any questions or suggestions or has an interest in organizing the Cancer Hot Line or Cancer Management Center locally, we will be happy to furnish assistance and information. Contact:

The Cancer Hot Line
4410 Main Street
Kansas City, MO 64111
816-932-8453

Glossary of terms in lay language

Benign. Cells forming a tumor that will not continue to grow and are not presently cancerous. They cannot spread from their original site and reach the bloodstream or lymphatic system.

Biopsy. The examination of tissue to determine whether it is malignant or benign.

Cancer. The uncontrolled growth of malignant cells.

Carcinogen. A cancer-causing substance.

Carcinoma. A malignant tumor arising in the sheets of cells covering the surface of the body and lining various glands.

Chemotherapy. The course of treatment through the use of chemicals.

Immunization therapy. The course of treatment by activating the immune system.

Leukemia. Cancer arising in the blood-forming cells of the bone marrow.

Lymphoma. Cancer arising in the lymph nodes.

Malignant. Cells which will continue to grow geometrically and are considered cancerous.

Metastasize. The breaking away of cancer cells from the original tumor, settling elsewhere in the body and forming a new tumor.

Nuclear medicine. Another term for scans or tomograms.

Oncologist. A doctor specializing in the treatment of cancer. He may further specialize in medicine, radiation or surgery, but always in relation to cancer.

Palliative treatment. Treatment that relieves pain and symptoms of disease but does not cure the disease.

Pathology. The examination of tissues and body fluids to determine whether malignant cells are present and to ascertain the type of cells.

Prognosis. The projected future course of the illness.

Protocol. A specific treatment or series of treatments that has been developed to treat cancer.

Radiotherapy. Treatment through the use of radiation or X rays.

Recurrence. The return of cancer in a different part of the body or the same part after it had been thought to be in remission or cured.

Remission. When cancer can no longer be found to be present but cannot be determined as cured.

Sarcoma. A malignant tumor arising in supporting structures, such as fibrous tissue and blood vessels.

Scan. A picture of a particular part of the body, such as brain, liver, or bones, produced by counting the radiation caused by radio-active substances injected to that part. A cat scan gives a detailed picture of a cross section of
the body.

Tomogram. A computer-produced vertical X ray capable of giving continuous "vertical slices" of various parts of the body.

Tumor. The mass caused by a concentration of cells, either benign or malignant.

Multidisciplinary second opinion centers

The following institutions have advised they will, when specifically requested, provide a multidisciplinary second opinion. This means that the patient is allowed to sit in front of a pathologist, diagnostic radiologist, surgeon, radiation oncologist, medical oncologist or other pertinent physicians. They hear their case discussed and are told all their options. **Be certain the patient specifically requests a multidisciplinary second opinion.** (Arranged geographically from East to West)

(*indicates free of charge)

Norris Cotton Cancer Center
Hanover, NH
Dr. O.R. McIntyre, Director
603-646-5505

Roger Williams Cancer Center
Providence, RI
Dr. Alan Weitberg, Director
401-456-2581

Montefiore Medical Center
Bronx, NY
Dr. Peter Wiernik, Associate Director
212-920-4826

Mount Sinai Cancer Center
New York City
Nana Miles
212-241-6368

Fox Chase Cancer Center
Philadelphia, PA
Ms. Julia Resnick
800-533-6784
215-728-2570 or

Johns Hopkins
Baltimore, MD
Mrs. Peggy Anderson
301-955-8964

Halifax Hospital
Daytona Beach, FL
Dr. Herbert Kerman, Director
904-254-4210

Regional Cancer Center Lourdes
Binghamton, NY
Dr. Robert Enck, Director of Oncology
607-798-5431

University of Rochester Cancer Center
Rochester, NY
Susan D. Smith, Assistant Director of Public Affairs
716-275-4911

Roswell Park
Buffalo, NY
Dr. Jerome Yates
716-845-3385

Ireland Cancer Center
Cleveland, OH
Dr. Nathan Berger, Director
216-844-8453

Ohio State University Hospitals
Columbus, OH
Nancy Brant
1-800-4-CANCER (Ohio)

Comp. Cancer Center/Met. Detroit
Detroit, MI
Dr. Michael Brennan, Director
313-833-0710

Loyola University
Chicago, IL
Dr. Richard Fisher
312-531-3336

Northwestern University
Chicago, IL
Dr. Leo Gordon
312-908-5284

University of Wisconsin Cancer Center
Madison, WI
Dr. Donald Trump
608-263-8600

St. Jude Childrens Research Hospital
Memphis, TN
(Children ONLY)
Dr. Joseph Simone, Director
901-522-0301*

University of Iowa Cancer Center
Iowa City, IA
Dr. Peter Jochimsen
319-356-3584

St. Vincent Cancer Center
Little Rock, AR
April Johnson
501-660-3900*

UTMB Cancer Center
Galveston, TX
Dr. Susan McClure, Director
409-761-1164

R.A. Bloch Cancer Management Center
Kansas City, MO
Bobbie Dall
816-932-8400*

Arizona Cancer Center
Tucson, AZ
Ms. Norma Maynard
601-626-6372

University of California, San Diego
San Diego, CA
Dr. Mark Green
619-294-6187

Cancer hot lines

Cleveland, OH
(216) 292-8222

Fort Lauderdale, FL
Broward (305) 721-7600
Dade (305) 547-6920

Fort Worth, TX
(817) 468-1660

Kansas City, MO
(816) 932-8453

Little Rock, AR
Local (501) 660-3900
Toll Free 1-800-632-4614

Pittsburgh, PA
(412) 782-4023

Comprehensive cancer centers

(listed alphabetically by state)

Univ. of Alabama Comprehensive Ca. Ctr.
1918 University Boulevard, Room 108
Birmingham, AL 35294
(205) 934-6612

Univ. of Arizona Ca Ctr.
1501 North Campbell Avenue
Tucson, AZ 85724
(602) 626-6372

Univ. of So. California Comprehensive Ca. Ctr.
Kenneth Norris Jr. Ca. Hospital and Research Inst.
1441 Eastlake Avenue
Los Angeles, CA 90033-0804
(213) 226-2370

Jonsson Comprehensive Ca. Ctr. (UCLA)
10-247 Factor Building
10833 Le Conte Avenue
Los Angeles, CA 90024-1781
(213) 825-8727

City of Hope National Med. Ctr.
Beckman Research Institute
1500 East Duarte Road
Duarte, CA 91010
(818) 359-8111, ext. 2292

Univ. of California at San Diego Ca. Ctr.
225 Dickinson Street
San Diego, CA 92103
(619) 543-6178

Northern California Ca. Ctr. (consortium)
1301 Shoreway Road
Belmont, CA 94002
(415) 591-4484

Univ. of Colorado Ca. Ctr.
4200 East 9th Avenue, Box B190
Denver, CO 80262
(303) 270-3019

Yale Univ. Comprehensive Ca. Ctr.
333 Cedar Street
New Haven, CT 06510
(203) 785-6338

Howard Univ. Ca. Research Ctr.
2041 Georgia Avenue, NW
Washington, DC 20060
(202) 636-7610 or 636-5665

Vincent T. Lombardi Ca. Research Ctr.
Georgetown Univ. Medical Center
3800 Reservoir Road, NW
Washington, DC 20007
(202) 687-2110

Papanicolaou Comprehensive Ca. Ctr.
Univ. of Miami Medical School
1475 Northwest 12th Avenue
Miami, FL 33136
(305) 548-4850

Illinois Cancer Council
36 South Wabash Avenue
Chicago, IL 60603
(312) 226-2371

Univ. of Chicago Ca. Research Ctr.
5841 South Maryland Avenue
Chicago, IL 60637
(312) 702-6180

Lucille Parker Markey Ca. Ctr.
University of Kentucky Medical Center
800 Rose Street
Lexington, KY 40536
(606) 257-4447

The Johns Hopkins Oncology Ctr.
600 North Wolfe Street
Baltimore, MD 21205
(301) 955-8638

Dana-Farber Ca. Institute
44 Binney Street
Boston, MA 02115
(617) 732-3214

Meyer L. Prentis Comp. Ca. Ctr. of Metro. Detroit
110 East Warren Avenue
Detroit, MI 48201
(313) 833-0710, ext. 429

Mayo Comprehensive Ca. Ctr.
200 First Street Southwest
Rochester, MN 55905
(507) 284-3413

Norris Cotton Ca. Ctr.
Dartmouth-Hitchcock Medical Center
2 Maynard Street
Hanover, NH 03756
(603) 646-5485

Memorial Sloan-Kettering Ca. Ctr.
1275 York Avenue
New York, NY 10021
1-800-525-2225

Columbia Univ. Ca. Ctr.
College of Physicians and Surgeons
630 West 168th Street
New York, NY 10032
(212) 305-6730

Roswell Park Memorial Institute
666 Elm Street
Buffalo, NY 14263
(716) 845-4400

Mt. Sinai School of Medicine
One Gustave L. Levy Place
New York, NY 10029
(212) 241-8617

Albert Einstein College of Medicine
1300 Morris Park Avenue
Bronx, NY 10461
(212) 920-4826

New York Univ. Ca. Ctr.
462 First Avenue
New York, NY 10016
(212) 340-6485

Univ. of Rochester Ca. Ctr.
601 Elmwood Avenue, Box 704
Rochester, NY 14642
(716) 275-4911

Duke Univ. Comprehensive Ca. Ctr.
P.O. Box 3843
Durham, NC 27710
(919) 684-6342 of (919) 286-5515

Lineberger Ca. Research Ctr.
Univ. of North Carolina School of Medicine
Chapel Hill, NC 27599
(919) 966-4431

Bowman Gray School of Medicine
Wake Forest Univ.
300 South Hawthorne Road
Winston-Salem, NC 27103
(919) 748-4354

Ohio State Univ. Comprehensive Ca. Ctr.
410 West 12th Avenue
Columbus, OH 43210
(614) 293-8619

Case Western Reserve Univ.
Univ. Hospitals of Cleveland
Ireland Cancer Center
2074 Abington Road
Celveland, OH 44106
(216) 844-8453

Fox Chase Ca. Ctr.
7701 Burholme Avenue
Philadelphia, PA 19111
(215) 728-2570

Pittsburgh Ca. Institute
230 Lothrop Street
Pittsburgh, PA 15213-2592
1-800-537-4063

Univ. of Pennsylvania Ca. Ctr.
3400 Spruce Street
Philadelphia, PA 19104
(215) 662-6364

Roger Williams General Hospital
825 Chalkstone Avenue
Providence, RI 02908
(401) 456-2070

St. Jude Children's Research Hospital
332 North Lauderdale Street
Memphis, TN 38101
(901) 522-0694

The Univ. of Texas
M.D. Anderson Ca. Ctr.
1515 Holcombe Boulevard
Houston, TX 77030
(713) 792-6161

Utah Regional Ca. Ctr.
Univ. of Utah Medical Center
50 North Medical Drive, Room 2C10
Salt Lake City, UT 84132
(801) 581-4048

Vermont Regional Ca. Ctr.
Univ. of Vermont
1 South Prospect Street
Burlington, VT 05401
(802) 656-4580

Massey Ca. Ctr.
Medical College of Virginia
Virginia Commonwealth Univ.
1200 East Broad Street
Richmond, VA 23298
(804) 786-9641

Univ. of Virginia Medical Ctr.
Box 334
Primary Care Center, Room 4520
Lee Street
Charlottesville, VA 22908
(804) 924-2562

Fred Hutchinson Ca. Research Ctr.
1124 Columbia Street
Seattle, WA 98104
(206) 467-4675

Wisconsin Clinical Ca. Ctr.
Univ. of Wisconsin
600 Highland Avenue
Madison, WI 53792
(608) 263-6872

Where to find answers

If you have questions concerning a specific type of cancer or where to get treatment, call the Cancer Information Service, a free service of the National Cancer Institute, on their toll-free number: 800-4CANCER.

By calling this number, you will automatically be routed to your local Cancer Information Service. If there is no Cancer Information Service in your area, it will automatically connect you with the National Cancer Information Service lines in Rockville, Maryland.

Request the state-of-the-art therapy for your type and stage of cancer. Also, request all current open protocols from everywhere in the United States for your specific type and stage of cancer. This will give you peace of mind knowing your doctor is giving you the best possible treatment. If you have any questions, ask your doctor.

About the authors

Richard A. (Dick) Bloch, born in Kansas City, Missouri on February 15, 1926, is the youngest of three sons.

An entrepreneur at heart, at age nine he bought a hand printing press and started a business. He was so successful that by his twelfth birthday he had progressed to three automatic presses and was doing much of the printing for all the high schools in Kansas City. After high school, he sold his business to a college in Iowa as a model shop for use in printing courses.

Dick attended the Wharton School of Finance at the University of Pennsylvania where he received a bachelor of science degree in economics. While in college, he bought cars, took them apart, put them back together and then sold them to pay for his expenses.

After graduation, Bloch worked for a brokerage firm in Kansas City, and after a short time, joined forces with his older brother, Henry, in the formation of the United Businesss Company, a firm offering small businessmen bookkeeping, management assistance, collection and income tax preparation services. The demand for tax preparation had become so great that in 1955 they started a new company specializing in tax preparation—H&R Block, Inc.—with Dick as chairman of the board. Today, they operate more than 9,000 offices worldwide and prepare over 10,000,000 returns annually.

Since Bloch's bout with cancer, he has focused his attention on working "to help the next person who gets cancer." He and his wife, Annette, created the Cancer Hot Line in Kansas City and are helping others start Hot Lines in their cities. They formed the R.A. Bloch Cancer Management Center, which they hope will act as a model for other communities to copy. An exciting project conceived by Bloch on which he is currently working with the NCI is called Protocol Data Query (PDQ). A computer service, available to any doctor, it will specify recommended treatments from the various cancer centers for every type of cancer.

In 1982, Dick was appointed by President Reagan to the National Cancer Advisory Board, whose purpose is to advise the director of the National Cancer Institute.

Annette Modell Bloch was born in Philadelphia, Pennsylvania where she lived until her marriage to Dick in 1946. She and Dick have three daughters—Barbara, Nancy and Linda, and seven grandchildren.

Her family always her top priority, Annette has also participated in many civic activities and is now Dick's partner in all of their cancer projects including public appearances and talks to various groups.

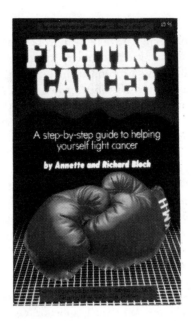

A step by step guide to help a patient help themselves fight cancer.

AVAILABLE FREE AT YOUR
LOCAL PUBLIC LIBRARY

If your library does not have Fighting Cancer or Cancer...there's hope, they may get 2 copies free postpaid by sending a request on their stationery to R.A. Bloch Cancer Foundation, Inc., 4410 Main St., Kansas City, Missouri 64111.

The first book is free to any cancer patient.

If you would like to order more copies of *Cancer...there's hope* or *Fighting Cancer*, please complete the following order form.

Cancer...there's hope is $3.00 including postage. *Fighting Cancer* is $4.00 including postage. Please use check or money order.

Please send me

_____ copies of *Cancer...there's hope*

_____ copies of *Fighting Cancer*

I enclose $ _____ *

Mr./Mrs./Miss _____

Address _____

City _____

State _____ Zip _____

Mail to: R.A. Bloch Cancer Foundation, Inc.
4410 Main Street
Kansas City, Missouri 64111

*This money will be used to assist cancer patients.

notes

notes

notes